HOUSING AND HEALTH

Housing and Health

The Relationship between Housing Conditions and

the Health of Council Tenants

D. S. BYRNE
S. P. HARRISSON
J. KEITHLEY
P. McCARTHY
University of Durham

Gower

Published by

Gower Publishing Company Limited,
Gower House,
Croft Road,
Aldershot,
Hants GU11 3HR
England

Gower Publishing Company,
Old Post Road,
Brookfield
Vermont 05036
USA

British Library Cataloguing in Publication Data

   Housing and health : the relationship between
   housing conditions and the health of council
   tenants.
   1. Public housing——Great Britain   2. Public
   health——Great Britain
   I. Byrne, David, *1947-*
   363.5'8   HD7288.78.G7

ISBN: 0 566 00864 5

Printed in Great Britain

Contents

List of tables

List of figures

1 Housing and health: the historical context

These evils, and the misery consequent upon them,
is (sic) much increased by peculiar faults in the
form and construction of the humble dwellings of
the poorer classes. (*Select Committee on the Health
of Towns*, 1840, p.viii)

INTRODUCTION

Policy and practice with regard to housing and health can be
seen as having gone hand in hand in this country for a period
of approximately one hundred years : that is to say from the
recognition in the 1840s of the public health problems occas-
ioned by housing conditions as part of the life experience of
the urban working class, until the major development of 'mass
housing' in the 1950s. An account of these historical developments is of the greatest importance in providing a basis for
understanding the health consequences of housing in the 1980s.
In subsequent chapters in this book it will be seen that the
'unhealthy housing' of the 1980s consists in the large part of
two elements of the housing stock, a) that constructed in the
1930s in the aftermath of the first major effective slum clearance legislation in this country, which was specifically directed at improving the health of slum dwellers by improving their
housing conditions, and, b) that constructed in the 'mass

housing' boom of the late 1950s to early 1970s in a period
when health considerations seem to have disappeared from the
agenda of items to be considered in framing a housing policy.

The purpose of this chapter is to trace the relationship between housing and health in urban England from the beginning
of the nineteenth century to the present day. It will be both
chronological and thematic in form. The chronology will be
based upon the notion of broad and distinctive periods in the
last hundred years which can be distinguished, very crudely,
in terms of the major focus of housing-health policy. These
are:

1830s-1860s : The period of the recognition of the nature of
the health problems of an urbanising society in general, and
of the relationship between housing conditions and health outcomes in particular.

1860s-1890 : The period of development of state regulation of
a private system of housing provision - a) with regard to the
quality control of construction, and b) with regard to the
elimination of the worst individual elements of existing provision.

1890-1919 : The aftermath of the 1890 Housing of the Working
Classes Act - the emergence of organised working class demands
for state housing provision and real slum clearance.

1919-1939 : The development of state housing - large scale
provision with large scale clearance ; 'homes fit for heroes'
versus 'sanitary adequacy'.

1939-1955 : War and its housing consequences - 'homes fit for
heroes' happens.

1955-mid 1970s : Slum clearance without health.

This chapter will be constructed around these periods. In
the discussion of each period a set of themes will be pursued
and will comprise the following. Firstly, the nature of the
understanding of the relationship between housing conditions
and health outcomes which was displayed in each of these
periods; this will be referred to as the 'social epidemiology
of health and housing'; secondly, the contribution of the
'social epidemiology of health and housing' to the formation
of housing policy. In considering the relationship between
the understanding of the health consequences of housing and
the formation of housing policy, two dimensions are used. The
first is that which is the traditional concern of historians
of these matters, namely, the way in which scientific

understanding influenced the development of understanding among the political/administrative elite in a fashion which led to policy developments. The second dimension is that of class action. Concern with the first dimension typifies the focus of the work of A.S. Wohl as reviewed by John Foster (1979) :

> However agreeably, we quickly find ourselves drawn
> into the concerned discourse of the upper class.
> This discourse, built upon a wealth of administrative
> experience, scientifically substantiated and learning
> its own lessons, necessarily provides for itself,
> within the changing balance of its own debates,
> complete explanations for each stage of the legislative
> process. We tend to forget, not from any deliberation,
> but from the lack of alternatives, that the completeness
> of these examinations is, of course, illusory. (p.49)

This dimension might be characterised as being the recognition by the state, in the form of the administrative/political elite which directs the operations of the state, of the problems for the reproduction of labour power posed by urban housing conditions. Consequent policy can be interpreted as the executive action by the state, functioning with regard to the collective interests of capital in order to resolve these problems.

However, in the period after 1890 at least (and possibly before, but the groundwork of investigation is grossly incomplete), the historian has always to remember the importance of active, conscious, organised working class action on housing issues. In this context the contribution of 'social epidemiology of housing and health' to the formation of working class political culture is of particular interest. Of clear and direct significance is the general understanding of the relationship between the occurrence of tuberculosis and poor housing conditions which informed working class political action on housing in the first half of this century. Thus the second dimension is that of class action.

Consideration of housing policy after 1890 always has to be concerned with the outcome of the conflict between these two dimensions; the desire of the capitalist system to ensure its own reproduction (the functionalist element), and the demands of an organised working class for reforms which could well, if met in full, be dysfunctional for that same system (the action element).

The foregoing paragraphs will have provided some clues about a general perspective which informs this chapter in particular and the book in general, i.e. the way in which the development

of urban forms as a result of the development of the capitalist mode of production has had consequences for health or, as
Doyal puts it, 'the social production of health and illness'
(1979). To quote again from Doyal (1979):

> This is not to suggest that the physical and chemical
> laws governing disease mechanisms can be simply aban-
> doned, but rather that they must be seen to operate
> within a social and economic context which is
> constantly changing. (p. 47)

This chapter is about the course of changes. The final
theme to be pursued is that of the health consequences of housing policies, which is the subject matter of the study reported as the major part of this book. The chapter will take the
form of an historical review concerned to a very considerable
extent with the health outcomes of the absence of housing
policy: with the way in which the housing provided without any
regulations in the early nineteenth century, festered as a
locale of ill health and as a causal factor in ill health
until the 1930s. However, the absence of policy, laissez-
faire, is itself a policy of sorts, and from the 1860s onwards
the consequences of active policy can be observed through the
eyes of contemporaries. Indeed, it was such observation
which in the interwar years served as the basis of what might
be regarded as the finest flowering of the social epidemiology
of health and housing in all its aspects.

A range of good secondary texts is available on national
housing policy (National Community Development Project, 1977;
Merrett, 1979; Melling, 1980; Dunleavy, 1981), but most of
the studies specifically orientated towards the relationship
between housing and health, carried out as they were by
Medical Officers of Health, consist of local investigations.
There is general agreement among historians of housing that
the local dimension is of crucial importance with regard both
to the recognition of the nature of the housing problem and
to the determination of the nature of housing policy in
practice (e.g. see Melling, 1980). The study which will be
reported in subsequent chapters of this book focuses on
council housing in the Metropolitan District of Gateshead.
It was thus thought to be most appropriate to consider in this
chapter the rich vein of local material on Gateshead and, as
far as possible therefore, a local dimension relating to
Tyneside in general and Gateshead in particular has been
included in the historical review.

.. in a word, we must confess that in the working-
men's dwellings of Manchester, no cleanliness, no
convenience, and consequently no comfortable family
life is possible; that in such dwellings only a
physical degenerate race, robbed of all humanity,
degraded, reduced morally and physically to best-
iality, could feel comfortable and at home. (Engels,
1892/1958, p.63)

The character of urban life in the first half of the nineteenth century in the United Kingdom has been fully described,
both by contemporary observers in the production of the Blue
Book Inquiries which, together with his own direct observation,
were the basis of Engels' denunciation, and in a range of
subsequent historical works of which Enid Gauldie's *Cruel
Habitations* (1974) is a particularly relevant example.
Gateshead was no exception. Robert Rawlinson in his report of
1850 asserted :

...neither plan nor written description can
adequately convey to the mind the true state and
condition of the room-tenements and of the inhabitants occupying them. The subsoil on the sloping side
of the hill is damp and most foul, the brickwork of
the buildings is ruinous, the timber rotten ; and
an appearance of general decay pervades the whole
district. (Quoted in Manders, 1974, p. 63)

The 'social epidemiology of health and housing' which was
associated with this was clearly understood by six local
doctors who wrote a report on the health of Gateshead in 1849
and submitted it to Rawlinson (who was Superintending Inspector
of the Board of Health) who reproduced it in his report. They
included a lengthy description of dwellings in Gateshead,
including those 'most recently created' and concluded:

Any one visiting these localities cannot be
surprised that they are generally severely visited
by disease at all times of the year .(Rawlinson, 1850;
quoted in Manders 1974, p.182)

Of course investigations of this sort did not differentiate
in any very precise fashion between housing conditions on the
one hand and inadequate or non-existent drainage and general
nuisances on the other. Gauldie (1974) has referred,

critically, to this:

> The paradox we have to deal with is that the
> public health movement is at the same time an
> important part of the history of housing, and
> totally irrelevant to it. While it is true that
> attention to the subject of urban housing conditions
> was first drawn not by philanthropists but by those
> interested in public health it is also true that
> the treatment of housing as part of the public
> health problem instead of as a subject for separate
> economic study and political action is a chief
> reason for the failure to provide successful
> remedies. (p. 85)

The present authors do not agree. It was the problem of
cost, associated with the public health consequences of poor
housing, which led to any change in this period. Rawlinson
argued this locally as Chadwick (1842) had nationally and the
establishment of a local Board of Health in 1852 was, clearly,
largely a response to the very real problems of ensuring the
continued physical reproduction of the industrial working
class. It is important to remember the actual scale of this
problem. In Liverpool at the time, of all children born in
labourers' families 62 per cent were dead before the age of
five. Cities had never reproduced themselves, but in a
society that was predominantly urban, that mattered a great
deal more than it had in the past. Roger's (1971) account of
the response of Gateshead to the 1848 Act illustrates this
concern quite clearly.

Of particular significance here is the absence of any housing intervention in this period. Building by-laws were not
made in Gateshead until 1861 and it was not until after that
date that there was any housing purpose built for the working
class. Instead, the working class were accommodated by a
process of multi-occupation of dwellings built for the prosp-
erous. Of particular interest here is the way in which houses
in Barnes Close built in the 1830s and 1840s had been converted into tenement property in multi-occupation by the 1850s.
This locale and the estate that replaced it after slum clearance in the 1930s will be discussed later.

One point worth making about this period is the differential
impact of epidemic disease. Many popular texts report that a
major rationale behind Victorian public health measures was
that epidemics were no respectors of persons or higher social
classes. The evidence from Gateshead of the impact of cholera
in this period is quite otherwise, with the locations of
incidence of this disease and of fatalities from it being

clearly associated with poverty and poor housing conditions
(see Manders, 1974).

This section will conclude with a very brief discussion of
the nature of the epidemiological understanding of the
relationship between housing and health conditions in this
period. The prevailing orthodoxy was of a miasmic theory of
infectious disease - diseases were caused and transmitted by
bad smells. The observational basis of this was sound - where
the smells were, there the disease was also. Only in 1849 was
Snow to identify the water borne nature of cholera and the
distinctive nature of various 'fevers' was not fully recognised and even less often separately diagnosed. It is now
known that the miasmic theory was erroneous in relation to
ultimate causation but its policy consequences, which were
pressures for good ventilation in housing, for access for
rubbish collection, and for nuisance removal in general, were
remarkably beneficial. The miasmic theory was wrong about
what caused disease but it was not wrong about what predisposed people to get diseases. This was why state regulation of
construction standards was, to some considerable degree,
effective in improving conditions.

1860-1890: Regulation and prosperity

Housing built in Gateshead, and in much of the rest of Tyneside, between 1860 and 1910 includes a very large proportion
of Tyneside flats. This is a housing form unknown elsewhere
in the United Kingdom outside a very limited area in the East
End of London. What appears to be one rather large terraced
house has two front doors side by side and the building
contains two separate and self contained flats. In general,
the downstairs flat consists of three rooms plus scullery and
yard and the upstairs flat has four rooms, although in the not
infrequent three storied versions the upper flat will also
have two attic rooms. In Sunderland, the Tyneside flat is
relatively uncommon. Instead the predominant late nineteenth century housing form is the single storied terraced
cottage which is well described by Dennis (1972). In Belfast
one finds kitchen and parlour houses. Most British cities
have many streets of small, two storied, self contained
terraced houses - Coronation Street is typical. In Scottish
cities there are tenements instead; the red sandstone three,
four and five roomed dwellings in tenement blocks in Govan are
representative. Despite the fact that the typical Scots
form is called a tenement, it is very important to realise
that these are not what was generally meant by tenements in
the nineteenth century. Then, and now in England, a
tenement was a dwelling built for the affluent which had
been given over to multiple occupation. Some of the best

7

examples remaining are to be found in Dublin (see Byrne, 1984)
and the social ambiance is well expressed in many of O'Casey's
plays. In Gateshead the Barnes Close area was tenemented.
The reason for the very rapid degeneration of early nineteenth
century stock into tenements is easily outlined. This housing
was, overwhelmingly, built as a speculation in rents and the
rental income from it tenemented and multi-occupied, was often
greater than if it had been let to a middle class family.
Before the 1850s this was how the working class of cities was
housed - in multi-occupation in dwellings built for the higher
social classes.

Tyneside flats, Sunderland cottages, Coronation Street and
red sandstone tenements are different. These were built as
single family homes (sometimes, as in Belfast, they were built
to be shared by two households but this was not general) for
working class people. This was the first purpose built,
urban, working class housing built on a general scale. Why
the shift? Tyneside flats are actually rather small in
comparison with other examples of this sort of housing, largely because of the topography of Tyneside which made building
land very expensive and led to the development of a 'cram them
in' form of urban design, in contrast with neighbouring
Sunderland where land was cheaper and a single storey design
was adopted to minimise building costs. Nonetheless, they
were not all that small and are generally substantial, brick
built dwellings with good quality timber work, stone lintels
and sills and slated roofs. By the 1890s they were costing
about £250 per pair to construct (North Tyneside Community
Development Project, 1977; and local evidence to the Royal
Commission on the Housing of the Working Classes, 1885) and in
the Board of Trade Report on Rents, Wages and Prices (1908)
shows that their rents were high. Local rents in 1906 were as
shown in Table 1.1.

Table 1.1
Rents on Tyneside in 1906

1 room	2/6d
2 rooms in tenement	3/6d to 4/-
3 roomed flat	4/- to 5/3d
4 roomed flat	6/- to 7/-

(source: Board of Trade, 1908)

At this time in this area a skilled fitter earned 35/- a week, a bricklayer 39/7d in summer, a builder's labourer 23/- to 26/-, a shipyard labourer 22/-, a seaman 30/- and a docker 5/- a day. Miners earning 30/- to 40/- a week frequently received housing with the job, although this did not generally happen in the conurbation, as opposed to the surrounding parts of the coalfield.

What the 1906 figures show is the existence of a divided working class; a high waged, skilled group living in Tyneside flats and paying high rents and a low waged, non skilled group living in tenements at lower rents.

In fact it can be argued that it was high wages for some which was the origin of the purpose built working class housing, rather than legislative intervention by the local state in the form of by-laws. This may seem contradictory when the earlier statement about any dwelling always having a higher rent when multi-occupied as opposed to singly occupied is recalled, but the change in logic derives from the character of the development process in the second half of the nine-teenth century. The point at which large amounts of capital were required in the process of house building was in the first land purchase. Manders (1974) lists a string of Gateshead estate purchases of which the purchase of six acres of the Rabbit Banks Farm by William Affleck for £4,600 is typical. The process beyond this point has not been pursued in Gateshead but evidence for North Shields and Benwell shows that in those neighbouring locales the developer put in streets and services and sold off building plots to small builders. The uniformity of dwellings constructed was a consequence of the covenant attached to the plot sale which, as the deeds of the dwellings show, specified a particular quality and form of construction and usually asserted that the dwellings must be for single or not more than two families. Developers could never sell all their land in one go. An area of 27 acres in North Shields took 25 years to develop. The value of the land sold later was determined by what had been built on that sold earlier, hence the covenants.

It could well be argued that building by-laws (Gateshead's were described as 'exceptionally imperfect' by Dr F.W. Barry in 1884) which were the formal method of regulating construct-ion standards, were of less significance than the logic of developers' profits. However the by-laws became more strin-gent and insisted in particular on ventilation and cubic cap-acity of rooms. A series of national measures, in particular the Nuisances Removal Act of 1855, the Sanitary Act of 1866 and the Public Health Acts of 1848, 1867 and 1875, all contained elements which gave local authorities powers to regulate housing. As Gauldie (1974) comments:

> ... the idea of public health was acceptable
> where interference in housing was not... So
> it was that almost all legislation on housing
> up to 1875 fell within the health laws. (p. 140)

Clearly what was happening in Gateshead, as in other industrial towns and cities, was the result of a combination of
factors. High wages for skilled workers (real wages doubled
between 1850 and 1900) made working class housing a possibil-
ity. At the same time sanitary considerations produced by-
laws which required, however imperfectly, healthier housing.
The two came together in types of construction which Manders
(1974), after listing its defects, summarily identifies thus:

> It should be remembered, however, that these
> flats were immeasurably better than any
> dwellings for the working class in Gateshead
> which had hitherto existed. (p. 170)

The social epidemiology of housing and health takes two
forms in this period. On the one hand the sanitary understanding of earlier periods informed attempts at state regulation of the quality of new construction through by-laws. On
the other hand the new housing had health consequences which
were rapidly perceived and commented on by medical practitioners and others. Medical Officers' of Health Reports from the
1880s through until the 1930s compared health outcomes in the
tenements with those in the 'decent mean streets'. The public
health problem was that the bases of better health of the
flat dwellers, in housing as in other respects, were their
higher wages. This left the casually employed poor whose wage
levels were such as to preclude them from the better stock.

The only intervention in this period of any significance was
not that by the state, despite Acts in 1861, 1866 and 1885.
Rather it was 'philanthropic housing' best known in the form
of Peabody Buildings, and often described as 'philanthropy at
five per cent'. The intention was to build dwellings which
required a lesser return on capital, were of lower standard
than that provided by market forces for the aristocracy of
labour, and would therefore be available to the poor. There
were not many of these and Merrett (1979) after a summary of
evidence concludes that, generally, the poor did not get into
them because rent levels were still too high. None were built
in Gateshead although one large block, The Newcastle
Industrial Dwellings (now the Garth Heads Hall of Residence
for Newcastle Polytechnic) was built in the 1860s for quayside
dock labourers in Newcastle. These philanthropic bodies were

not able to function without state aid. Merrett (1979) comments that the Labouring Classes Dwelling Houses Act of 1866 was used almost exclusively by them. (This Act permitted the Public Works Loan Commissioners to provide finance to societies and trusts of this sort). Their importance lies not so much in the relatively little they did, as in the recognition of the necessity for assistance to the poor if they were ever to obtain sanitarily adequate housing.

1890-1919: The aftermath of the 1890 Housing of the Working Classes Act: the emergence of organised working class demands for housing

This period is not distinguished from that immediately preceding it because there was a new housing system created during it. That was not to happen until the inter war years. Rather it was characterised by a new politics of housing in which the representation of working class interests by working class people and political organisations assumed a new significance. The vehicle of the dispute was generally part III of the Housing of the Working Classes Act 1890 which allowed local authorities to supply housing directly for rent and which had to be adopted by the authority to take effect. Political campaigns about the use of this Act were a crucial mode through which the early Labour Party developed. This has been written about extensively elsewhere (see Byrne, 1980; 1982), but it is worth returning to the story to see the part that popular understanding of the 'social epidemiology of housing and health' played in it. Those in favour of the adoption of the Act were, usually, an alliance of local medical men and labour (the small 'l' is deliberate) representatives. In Gateshead Drs. Cox and Abrahams were representatives of the former, much supported by the leading Liberal figure, Robert Spence Watson, one of the authors of the Newcastle programme of the 1890s which moved that party in a radical direction. The labour representatives in Gateshead in the 1890s were solid trade union councillors although by 1910 in Gateshead, as elsewhere on Tyneside, the battles were generally fought by the avowedly socialist Independent Labour Party (ILP). The rejection of the 1899 effort to get part III of the 1890 Act adopted was due to factors well understood by the local *Gateshead Guardian* :

It is remarkable how some of the property
owners who have seats on the council look
askance at any suggestions in the direction
of remedying such an evil. One would think
they had some interest in prolonging this
undesirable state of affairs. One of the
best things that could happen to the council
would be for all the property holding
councillors and aldermen to be cleared out
for a couple of years. During the period
some good could be done and the nuisance of
overcrowding and unhealthy dwellings removed.
Alderman Hindmarsh (a prominent local estate
agent and landlord) draws largely upon his
imagination when he describes Gateshead as a
health resort. (20 January, 1900)

The character of the arguments which were to be repeated
over Tyneside in the years leading up to 1914 is revealing.   In
1913 when an effort was being made to get Tynemouth County
Borough Council to build housing, Alderman Coulson, a
prominent Tory builder and landlord, blamed the high death
rate in that borough on:

... the filth and dirt people live in. This is
the evil, not the condition of the houses.
Put some of these people into Alnwick Castle
and by the time they have been there one month
it will be a slum. (*Shields Daily News*, 5 October
1914)

When the issue was raised again in 1914 a local member of
the ILP wrote that:

The opposition will consist, Liberal and Tory
alike, of those who feel interested in preventing
the Corporation from building cheap and healthy
dwellings to compete with the highly rented
and unhealthy dwellings of themselves and their
friends. (North Tyneside CDP, 1977, p. 12)

The nature of the demands being made on the local authorities on Tyneside were specific, limited and health related.
They were for local state intervention in housing for the
poor to provide an alternative to the tenements. The argument was that economies of scale in the provision and the
elimination of the specific return of the housing landlord

would reduce the costs of provision to the point where the poor could afford the rent levels. It was for a municipal version of the philanthropic housing, not for the design and quality revolution associated with 'homes fit for heroes'. Many of the medical supporters, for example Abrahams, were social imperialists and eugenicists concerned with the impact of urban conditions on potential working class recruits to the forces and the quality of industrial labour in a competitive world. What seems to be new is the organised working class element in demands for the promotion of healthy housing. It was this factor which was to be most important in the post war period.

1919-1939: 'Homes fit for heroes' and homes for the poor.

> It was crucial for the ideological function of
> the housing programme that the houses be indis-
> putably better than the working class houses of
> the past. Housing on garden city lines was not
> only unmistakeably different from the usual forms
> of working class housing but it had also been
> regarded as beyond the means of working class
> incomes, and for that reason it was just what
> the government needed in order to validate its
> claim to the loyalty of the returning heroes.
> (Swenarton, 1981, p. 187)

The transformation which occurred in the housing of the working classes, or rather the housing of some of the working classes, in the immediate aftermath of the first world war is clearly visible. Swenarton (1981) fully documents the process which led to the provision of this stock and comments that local authorities concerned with public health criteria had this quality imposed upon them. Indeed, national and local evidence (see for example Byrne, 1980) illustrates clearly that housing built under the Addison Act of 1919 was the first built in the public sector in which health considerations were not the dominant factor and it was to be criticised for this throughout the interwar years, as was that constructed post 1924 under the Wheatley legislation. This housing was built to its extraordinarily high quality in response to strength. If there is any criticism of Swenarton's account it is that he does not fully recognise the extent to which the demand for 'cottage housing' had been part of the class pro-gramme since prewar days in Glasgow and had been generalised by Wheatley's campaigning.

Despite the high level of subsidy both the Addison Act and the Wheatley Act stock were too expensive for the poor. They

did have an impact on housing standards in the slums because
the movement of the aristocracy of labour from by-law housing,
the 'decent mean streets', into this stock left the former
available to poorer people. Wheatley had certainly understood
the dynamics of this process and overcrowding fell markedly
on Tyneside between 1921 and 1931. However, the main significance of this stock is its 'bench marking' effect. From 1919
to the present day the standard of good quality housing has
been judged, for owner occupation as well as public sector
renting, by the standard this stock set. In Gateshead some
dwellings of this quality were built between 1919 and 1931.
This introduced an additional element into the already highly
differentiated stock. For working class housing the hierarchy
established by 1930 was:

1) Good council housing

2) By-law housing

3) Council tenements

4) Multi-occupied tenements

   The element under 3), council tenements, is of particular
significance to the 'housing and health study'. By the early
1920s there was considerable opposition to the quality of the
new council housing and its consequent cost. In Tynemouth a
local Tory Councillor and general practitioner, Dr Harrison,
asserted that people wanted:

>   ... houses of two, three and four rooms - houses
>   which they could furnish and pay rent for. I
>   go about them in their homes and know exactly
>   what they want. (*Shields Daily News*, 27 September
>   1923)

   In Gateshead as in North Shields pressures of this sort led
to some small scale clearance under the 1890 Act and the building of some recently demolished flats. This was the beginning
of the process of differentiation in the provision of council
housing. One might say that council housing can be divided into two kinds, viz. that built when working class organisations
were strong and committed to good quality, and that built at
the initiative of the state in order to rectify problems of
health and quality of housing stock. The first kind closely
resembles, and is generally at least as good as and often better than, the quality of housing provided by market mechanisms
for lower middle class and working class owner occupation.
Much of the second kind was built between the late 1950s and
the early 1970s; part of it has been referred to as

'mass housing' (Dunleavy, 1981) and will be discussed later in
the chapter. There was a little of this built in the 1920s in
Gateshead. A lot of it dating from the 1930s is still in
existence, built in response to the first effective slum clearance legislation, the Greenwood Act of 1930. This Act imposed
a requirement on every authority with a population of more
than 20,000 to produce a general statement of its plans for
dealing with slum clearance and with the provision of more
houses in the following five years. It introduced subsidies,
additional to the existing Wheatley subsidies, on the basis of
per person rehoused in a clearance replacement scheme. The
intention was that the additional subsidies would, taken
together with falling building costs, bring the garden city
council housing in reach of the slum dwelling poor.

At the second reading of the Bill, Wheatley warned about the
likely outcome:

> Slumdom is inherent in the working-class dwellings
> of this country. The narrow streets, the damp
> conditions of the houses, the general sanitary
> defects of these dwellings, are all standing
> evidence that in the industrial development of
> this country we have come through an age of
> barbarism. We cannot leave out of account the
> fact that nearly every industrial centre in this
> country has its tens and hundreds of thousands of
> houses that are potential slums. It is no use
> approaching this question as if there were a
> given number of slums and that when we had dealt
> with them the problem was solved and we could
> turn to the next problem. It is a recurring
> factor and it will go on as long as we set aside
> for a particular section of the community an
> inferior quality of housing accommodation.
> (*Hansard*, 1929-30, vol. 237, p.2014)

The abolition of the Wheatley subsidies by the Housing (Financial Provisions) Act of 1933 ensured that there was, 'set
aside for a particular section of the community, an inferior
quality of housing accommodation'. In Gateshead this is very
well illustrated by the demolition of Barnes Close and the
transfer of its population to the Old Fold Estate which is one
of the 'housing and health'study areas. This will be documented in some detail, but before so doing the nature of the
technical understanding of the social epidemiology of housing
and health at this time will be considered.

Bradbury's *Casual factors in tuberculosis* (1933), a Tyneside
based study, provides a useful model. This was a comparative

study of Jarrow and Blaydon, two Tyneside urban districts with
approximately equal populations but very different tuberculosis death rates. The study is of very great interest not
just in an historical sense but because many of the methodological problems Bradbury dealt with recur in the study
reported in the present book. Bradbury did have one advantage
- a clearly defined dependent variable, viz. the occurrence in
a family of clinically diagnosed tuberculosis, but the logic
of his study closely resembled the 'housing and health' study.
As he said on causes:

> In a sense of course, there is only one cause of
> tuberculosis - the tubercle bacillus - and when
> in this report the various conditions studied are
> referred to as causes of tuberculosis they are
> understood as meaning conditions which favour the
> occurrence of tuberculosis in any way eg. by
> facilitating the entry of the tubercule bacillus
> into the body or by encouraging its proliferation
> within the body. (p.16)

Bradbury had two kinds of causal problems to sort out. One
was the problem of order: in this instance, most importantly,
whether poverty caused tuberculosis by facilitating the
disease or whether tuberculosis caused poverty by reducing the
capacity to engage in waged work. He resolved his order problem by consultation of case notes supplemented by direct
enquiry. He tried to establish chronological precedence in
order to establish causal ordering and concluded that poverty
caused tuberculosis. Equally, he had the problem of disentangling which factors did cause tuberculosis when poverty was a
multiple complex of possibly relevant factors. In particular
he tried to establish, by the use of relatively simple statistical techniques, if undernourishment and overcrowding were
each important or whether the association between the incidence of tuberculosis and either of the two factors mentioned
was due to a spurious association. Although this problem is
now dealt with using more complex techniques (especially log-
linear models) than the simple difference of proportion tests
used by Bradbury, the logic of modelling he employed closely
resembles the modelling used in the 'housing and health' study.
Figure 1.1 illustrates some possible relationships among
poverty, overcrowding and tuberculosis with the priority of
the first two to the third established by chronological ordering.

Model 1) says that the only way in which poverty causes
tuberculosis is through overcrowding. Model 2) says that
poverty causes tuberculosis through overcrowding and in other
ways. Model 3) says that poverty causes tuberculosis and

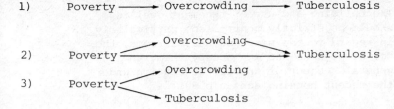

Figure 1.1 Three variable models

poverty causes overcrowding but that there is no relationship between overcrowding and tuberculosis.

   Bradbury's conclusion about the aetiology of tuberculosis in urban Tyneside in the 1930s was stated as follows:

> ... it is apparent that the association of tuber-
> culosis with poverty is of greater importance than
> with any of the other conditions studied. This
> is a very natural finding for as the whole is
> greater than the part, so is poverty of greater
> importance than the numerous conditions which
> accompany or result from it. The possible causes
> of the observed association between poverty and
> tuberculosis have been fully considered, and it
> has been shown that the chief element of this
> association is that poverty causes tuberculosis,
> rather than that tuberculosis leads to poverty.
> The principal means by which poverty is found to
> cause T.B. are the overcrowding and under-nourishment
> which are the chief distinguishing features
> between the poor and not poor families in the areas
> studied. (p.96)

   In Bradbury's two areas the percentage of deaths caused by tuberculosis were 13.2 per cent in Jarrow and 9.3 per cent in Blaydon (which was close to the United Kingdom average of 9.5 per cent). Since tuberculosis killed children and young adults it was the major cause of premature death. Anyone with any contact with that generation of people brought up in work-ing class Tyneside in the 1920s and 1930s, a generation which saw the death of many of its members from tuberculosis, is well aware of the profound impact this had on their lives and cultural and political attitudes. Work like Bradbury's demonstrated that the 'white plague' was not accidental - it was a disease of poverty and poor feeding and bad housing. When Bradbury made recommendations for the reduction of the incidence of the disease on Tyneside his first was:

1) The building and use of tenement dwellings
   should be strictly controlled, particularly
   in regard to the size and no. of rooms, the
   no. of persons who may occupy them, and the
   general subject of special regulation under
   the recent housing acts. (p.99)

Bradbury's work was of course not unique. It was merely an
important local instance of a variety of studies, many of
which are cited in the useful bibliography to A.E. Martin's
article on, *Environment, Housing and Health* (1967). The
evidence was often complex. M'Gonigle's work in Stockton
(1933), although subsequently disputed, seemed to demonstrate
negative consequences of rehousing for the slum cleared. This
was a consequence of a poorer diet when a larger proportion of
income had to be devoted to rent. Disentangling the different
effects of poverty, and indeed deciding whether such a
disentangling is appropriate, is a problem. The 1930s were a
period of major epidemiological investigation of the social
factors causal to ill health and one of the key factors
identified was housing. Indeed in the 1930s the local logic
of housing policy was about the relief of ill health as a
first priority. To see how this worked out it is useful to
look at the clearance procedure under the 1930 Act in
Gateshead.

At any time the existing housing stock is of far greater
significance for housing provision than any additions that can
be made to it in the short term. A possible impression that
may have been made by the first part of this section requires
correction here. The Wheatley and Addison Act housing was
important, but as late as the early 1960s the largest element
in the housing stock of places like Gateshead was that part
of it which had been built before the first world war. In
fact this had not been neglected in the 1920s. The first
thing that the first Gateshead Labour controlled council did
was to introduce a system of waterborne sewage disposal to
replace the earth and ash closet system in existence. The
scheme had been demanded since the 1880s. In 1911 the Medical
Officer of Health (MOH) had commented in his annual report:

In addition to manure heaps, the ash closets and
ashpits played an important part for the continual
fluid condition of these receptacles during hot
weather, when the quantity of ashes available for
de-ordorisation is diminished, gives the necessary
state, together with heat, for the rapid multiplication
of flies, which in turn invade the houses with feet

covered with filth to contaminate whatever food
they chance to drop upon. There can be no doubt,
notwithstanding that the tenements show up badly,
that the W.C. system throughout the town would
greatly improve matters during hot weather. (Quoted
in Gateshead Labour Party and Trades Council;
undated).

In 1923 when Labour gained control of the authority they,
against the opposition of private landlords, took on 200
employees in a direct labour scheme and converted 18,706
dwellings to a waterborne system in two years and four months.
This was, of course, in part an exercise in employment creat-
ion, but its health effects were major.

The conversion scheme applied to the whole town where required (i.e. to three-quarters of all dwellings). The main
slum removal of the 1920s was in fact a consequence of the
construction of the New Tyne Bridge built at this period, but
in the 1930s a major slum clearance programme was instituted.
Here tuberculosis was very important. Successive Gateshead
MOHs' Reports remarked on the effect of housing, for example:

> ... to cure cases in the small houses is impossible,
> to expect to prevent infection is equally impossible,
> unless the houses are properly constructed, and
> provision made for efficient ventilation. (1912,
> p.21)

> 92.3% of cases of TB are to be found in houses
> of four or less rooms. (1930, p.3a)

> One hopes that the big drive which is being made
> in slum clearance will bear fruit in the not too
> distant future in a reduction of the incidence of,
> and mortality from, Tuberculosis. (1933, p.40)

The first area represented under the 1930 Act was Barnes
Close built for the middle class in the 1830s and tenemented
slums by the 1850s. This area was occupied by poor people.
The MOH had commented in the 1912 Report:

> The class of people found in these dwellings
> consists in the main of the labouring and itinerant
> classes, who can ill afford to pay big rents.
> It is certainly true that we have in other parts
> of the town a considerable number of empty houses,
> but the rents are far beyond the paying powers of
> the people here concerned to occupy them. (p.43)

A full verbatim record of the enquiry is available. The MOH
described the Barnes Close area. It consisted of 203 dwellings
with 1,123 rooms housing 661 separate families comprising
2,652 persons; 333 families comprising 1,138 persons lived in
single rooms; 244 families comprising 1,123 persons lived in
two rooms; 97 families of more than five persons lived in
single rooms. In the year 1931 there were 1,840 cases of
tuberculosis in Gateshead i.e. 14.87 per 1,000 population. In
Barnes Close there were 90 i.e. 33.93 per 1,000 population. The
area had been the location of a cholera epidemic in 1854 and of
a typhus epidemic in 1910.

Most of the general cross examination, as opposed to cross-
examination relating to the conditions of individual dwellings,
was about this overall medical evidence. Dr Clayton, the MOH,
was cross examined extensively by Dr Charlesworth (his doctor-
ate was in civil law), a barrister who figured in a lot of
1930s inquiries in Tyneside. The burden of Charlesworth's
approach was: could poor nutrition be the cause of the
tuberculosis rather than the housing, and in any event 90 cases
and 10 deaths was a small number from which to generalise. The
MOH stood his ground and, as was almost invariably the case at
this time, (see North Tyneside CDP, 1977), the compulsory
purchase order was approved.

The estate built to replace Barnes Close at Old Fold was the
major housing replacement development of the 1930s. There were
482 dwellings of which about 10 per cent were flats. The
total cost per dwelling was £406 in contrast to £467 for the
188 houses built at Field House Lane. The difference in
standards between Wheatley and Greenwood Act housing was much
less in Gateshead than, for example, in North Tyneside (see
Byrne, 1980) where flats replaced houses but the 15 per cent
cut in costs did represent a major cut in standards, princip-
ally in relation to site densities. Between 1933 and 1939,
1,684 families were rehoused but at the outbreak of war only
half of the slum clearance programme had been completed. In
1942 there were 5,620 people living in property which had
been scheduled for demolition as part of the prewar clearance
programme.

In summary the inter-war period can be regarded as the beginning of a modern housing system. More than 5,000 new dwellings
were built in Gateshead in this period, divided into about 60
per cent private and 40 per cent council. Of those built for
the private sector the overwhelming majority were for owner
occupation, although in the late 1930s there was a small scale
revival of the building of Tyneside flats for rent. Private
renting was to remain the dominant tenure into the postwar

years but by the outbreak of war the new housing system of
owner occupation and council renting was fully developed. In
the public sector the contrast between good quality stock and
that built in order to replace slum cleared dwellings was
already evident. The result was the perpetuation within the
public sector of the existing division in private rented stock
between the purpose built housing in terraced flats inhabited
by the respectable working class and the tenements occupied
by the poor. Although Old Fold is rather less inferior to
its predecessors than is normally the case with the slum clearance estates of the 1930s, it has always been a segregated
locale. Indeed in many respects its remote and rather
unpleasant location close to factories isolated from other
residential areas is one of the major factors leading to its
low status.

The inter-war period saw a very fully developed medical and
political understanding of the social epidemiology of
housing and health. There was a considerable body of research
which fed directly into the national and local formation of
policy, particularly through the powerful role of Medical
Officers of Health. Also significant was the general popular
understanding of the unnecessary character of so much morbidity and mortality and of the potential for improving the
situation through housing provision. Indeed the existence of
a local authority housing system meant that housing had a
direct political potential as an agency for change with regard
to the social factors underlying poor health. This was much
more remote in the case of the financial aspects of poverty
which were derivatives of the wage system. At the outbreak
of war housing was an issue, throughout the war it remained
an issue, and at the end of the war it continued to be an
issue. This was in no small part, although by no means
entirely, because of the health potential of good housing.

*1939-1955: War and its housing consequences - 'Homes fit for
heroes' happens*

> It is worthwhile to re-emphasise that the solution
> of the housing problem will confer much more good
> on the community than the complete fulfilment of
> the National Health Service Act (MOH of Gateshead,
> *Annual Report for 1947*, quoted in *Gateshead Post*,
> 29 October, 1948)

With little bomb damage in Gateshead the authority found
itself in 1945 with the same housing stock it had had in 1939,
albeit a stock dilapidated by an almost complete absence of

repair. What was different was the character of the demands
for new housing, demands most powerfully and forcefully expressed by new households formed by discharged ex-servicemen and
women and by other war workers. And it was a demand for houses
- not flats. Despite efforts by architects to sell the concept
of flats, there was a commitment to high quality construction.
This was expressed by the Minister responsible, Aneurin Bevan,
when he asserted that he would be judged by contemporaries in
terms of the number of houses built, but by later generations
in terms of the quality of houses built, and he intended to be
judged by the criterion of the future. The national developments are fully documented elsewhere (eg. in Merrett, 1979).
Local attitudes in Gateshead were typified by Councillor
Armstrong, the Labour Chairman of the Housing Committee, when
rejecting a Rent and Ratepayer (i.e. anti labour local coali-
tion) proposal to build three and four storey flats instead
of houses. He asserted that in East Gateshead:

> ...people were just as much entitled to a garden
> and the amenities of two storey houses as anyone
> else. (*Gateshead Post*, 6 October 1948)

Nonetheless even at this early date there were pressures
which were to gather force in the early 1950s. Gateshead
County Borough (the urban core of the present Gateshead
Metropolitan Borough Council) was very short of land and had
not completed its pre-1939 slum clearance programme. The MOH
continuously returned to the problems this caused. Although
more than 2,000 good quality houses had been built by 1954
the pressure on the local authority was still considerable and
there had been very little progress with the slum clearance
programme. In fact the land problem was, to some considerable
degree, resolved by overspill building in the area of Felling
Urban District Council, but the major redirection in national
policy after 1954 had a dramatic local impact. Merrett (1979)
summarised this in terms of 1) a restriction of output to
300,000 dwellings per year in total, 2) the making of new
housebuilding for general needs, the preserve of the private
sector, 3) control of local authority output so that it was
confined to making up the private sector shortfall and 4):

> ... large scale housing renewal was to be
> stimulated, but in a particular framework.
> Repair, improvement and the conversion of the
> existing privately owned stock was to be
> encouraged by grants and by permitting rent
> increases tied to improvement... Housing renewal
> by means of clearance was to be the preserve of
> the local authorities : they 'should be encouraged

in future to concentrate their main housing
efforts on slum clearance and overspill building which only they can tackle effectively'
(p. 248) (internal quotation, *Ministry of Housing
and Local Government Report for the year 1955;*
1956, p.3)

This was the national direction towards mass housing which is
the subject of the next section of this chapter.

The immediate postwar period has been dealt with very
briefly but its importance is immense. It is the only period
in which the provision of local authority housing was the
normal method cf providing new houses. The symbolic dropping
of 'for the working classes' from legislation was an indicat-
ion that policy in this period intended the great majority of
new households to enter the council sector. It was the
abandonment of this commitment and the assertion that 'owner
occupation' was in future to be the 'normal' way of getting
a house which marked the change in policy in 1954. There are
two issues here. One is particular to council housing. This
postwar period saw the building of a large amount of very
good housing indeed in terms of design, construction standard,
location and layout. It consisted overwhelmingly of semi-
detached houses on garden city estates. Insofar as this and
the Addison and Wheatley Act housing of the inter-war years
is available in the council housing stock, it provides a means
of access through non market mechanisms to high quality housing. This access was historically complicated by rent levels
but is now largely independent of this factor. Thus, in
principle, poor people can get good housing because this stock
exists and is available to them. The implications of this
will be discussed in the methodological section.

The general issue is fundamental to the politics of housing
in Britain up to the present day. The assertion in policy
and elsewhere that owner occupation was to be the normal way
of getting a house meant that council housing acquired, at
least in national context, the status of a residual sector for
those who could not get a dwelling any other way. This issue
had been fought out in the inter-war years but was not resolved. In 1945-1951 it was resolved in favour of council housing as the normal tenure. Post 1954 things have gone the other
way, although until the 1980 Housing Act and the consequent
forced sale of council housing this was much less so in the
North East than in other parts of the United Kingdom (except
Scotland). The 'right to buy' under the 1980 Act is the
culmination of this process and the topic will be returned to
in the conclusion to this book. What is important about the

23

years after the second world war is that they were different.

1955-1974: Slum Clearance without consideration of health

> ...mass housing - large flatted estates of uniform
> housing quite distinct in form from the kinds of
> housing provided by market mechanisms. (Dunleavy,
> 1981, p.1)

The 1957 Housing Act was the major legislative initiative
concerned with slum clearance in the postwar period. Interestingly the Act displaced direct reference to health and
substituted 'not reasonably suitable for occupation' with
regard to the determination of the unfitness of individual
dwellings (section 4). However, section 42 which dealt with
area clearance referred to areas which:

> ...are unfit for human habitation, or are by reason
> of their bad arrangements, or the narrowness or bad
> arrangement of the streets, dangerous or injurious
> to the health of the inhabitants of the area...
> (section 42)

Cullingworth (1966) commented on this:

> These areas of bad arrangement...only come within
> the literal scope of the legislation if it can be
> shown that the health of the inhabitants is likely
> to be affected. This is virtually impossible to
> do in a literal sense today... (p. 180)

What is certain is that postwar public enquiries dealing
with slum clearance were much less impressive than their 1930s
precursors and that the social epidemiology of housing and
health played a far smaller part, if indeed any part at all,
in their proceedings. Even the orientation of the MOH with
regard to objectives was changing. In 1963 Gateshead's MOH
justified the continuation of the slum clearance programme
in very different terms from those which had been used as
recently as the late 1940s:

> ...it is by the clearance of these dwellings,
> now obsolete, decrepit and sometimes even ruinous
> that the wide spaces are found to make possible
> the potentially valuable commercial and business
> developments as well as the modern road improve-
> ments. (*Gateshead Post*, 29 November 1963)

There was not even a citation of health. Instead the
MOH was using the language of the commercial centre redevelop-
er and the inter-urban transport planner. This was the period
when in the words of one disillusioned local planner (the late
James Alder) whose orientation was somewhat eccentric for his
times, Gateshead was turned from a town into a road island.
Actually, Gateshead had begun building city centre flatted
blocks in the mid 1950s for reasons justified locally in terms
of land shortage, e.g.:

> Slum clearance necessitated the construction of
> houses for the displaced tenants and within the
> existing borough the resort to the building of
> multi-story flats for the working classes has
> been necessary. (*Gateshead Post*, 29 November
> 1963)

Merrett (1979) identifies a 'density bias' as above, and a
production bias which:

> ...took two forms. In the first place, the train-
> ing of architects does not create within them the
> self-image of a building worker with a specific
> set of design skills, which is what the majority
> are and must be, but the self-image of the artist
> genius whose sculpted forms soar above the urban
> landscape. Development gave the architects a
> free hand to attempt to stamp their greatness
> in the concrete form of a set of dwellings.
> Rehabilitation could only constitute the expression
> of a set of skills which in appearance
> were mundane. In the second place we know that
> rehabilitation work, with its heavy reliance on
> traditional craft labour, tends to be carried out
> by small contractors and by direct labour,
> whereas only large firms handle redevelopment
> contracts. So it has always been in the economic
> interest of the latter to push for clearance. (p. 122)

Add in competition for central sites and it can be realised
why, even for the MOH, health took a back seat.

The process whereby 'mass housing' became the public sector
urban form is beautifully described by Dunleavy (1981). Of
especial interest is his comment when reviewing professional
attitudes to this, that:

> The attitudes of the professions involved in the
> social aspects of housing were in general slightly

more ambiguous than those of the design
professions. Public Health Inspectors as
a body persistently pressed for radical action
on slum clearance, for the comprehensive
treatment of areas of bad housing, and for
quick solutions to rehousing problems. But,
in the early postwar period at least, they
were also opposed to very high density schemes
which had in the past been associated with
ill-health, and to tenement blocks in particular
... By the end of the decade, however, these
attitudes were voiced less and less frequently.
The undercurrent of disquiet about high-rise
amongst some social workers and doctors only
began to be noticed very late in the 1960s.
(pp. 138-139)

Mass housing in Gateshead will be documented by reference to
the background to the development of one of the estates in
which the 'housing and health' survey was conducted -
St Cuthberts Village. Unlike Nursery Lane in Felling which
has an extraordinary history of corruption in addition to its
design and construction problems, St Cutherts is a straightforward example of the general processes by which mass housing was imposed on public sector tenants. The first plan for
the construction of housing on this difficult site were
produced in the middle of the 1960s when the area was in the
process of being cleared. The press discussion at this time
refers continuously to land shortages as the reason for
building in this locale and the proposal was extensively reviewed as an example of new technically innovative architect-
ural practice. The principal architect responsible was quoted
as saying, "It is not exactly a tourist attraction now, but
it will be before long". (*Northern Echo*, 5 June, 1965).

The development was plagued with difficulties from the
beginning. At this time central government applied a 'cost
yardstick' to council house building. This was a ceiling
price per unit and, although it could be exceeded, it
operated to set a constraint on quality. The yardstick could
be amended to allow for difficult sites but the St Cuthberts
development was also at its cost limit in pure construction
terms. Initial estimates in 1964 were for £4,400 per three
bedroomed dwelling compared with £3,600 in conventional
eqivalents built on ordinary sites. The crucial consequence
of this yardstick was the decision in 1967 to install ceiling electric heating in the maisonettes, as the cheapest space
heating system in capital cost terms, without thought for the
implications for the people who were going to live in the

26

dwellings and pay the running costs.

The estate was completed by 1970 and was opened by the then
Prime Minister,Harold Wilson early in that year.It was criticised from the very beginning. In January 1970 the *Sunday Sun*
quoted a 'partner in Gateshead's oldest established firm of
private architects' to the effect that :

> ...the whole development looks 'unreal and dead'.
> I am firmly against the concept of shoving up
> these concrete blocks and cramming people in to
> live on top of each other... The tenants who are
> living there have found themselves in the middle,
> not of a dream but a nightmare. (11 January, 1970)

This article went on to quote from tenants who described the
dwellings as 'egg boxes' and rabbit hutches', although when
Wilson opened the estate in April 1970 he described it as an
example of the finest town planning in Europe.

Early complaints were dismissed as being to do with the
consequences of site works but by November 1971 a survey conducted by a resident demonstrated that more than half the
residents wanted to leave. The major local evening paper, the
Evening Chronicle carried an extensive investigation of the
situation in December 1971, only 18 months after the first
residents moved in, which concluded :

> St Cuthberts Village should never have been built.
> It is the wrong size, the wrong shape and in the
> wrong place. (30 December 1971)

From then on things got worse. A massive increase in real
terms in electricity charges made the dwellings impossible to
heat. They suffered from massive condensation problems with
amazing levels of fungal infestation. The last sentence is
meant literally. One of the research workers will never
forget being shown, in the mid 1970s, curtains in a
St Cuthberts maisonette with what appeared to be toadstools
growing on them, helping the tenant hang new ones, and returning a week later to be shown a fresh crop! The estate
appeared in the Department of the Environment Housing
Development Directorate's study of 'difficult to let' estates
(1980b) following on a decade of tenants' protests and tenants'
abandonment. In the late 1970s an intensive management
scheme was introduced and, most recently, a decision has been
taken to demolish a large part of the estate. However it has
been there for fifteen years. A lot of people have lived
there in housing introduced to replace the slums which, in

many respects, is an even worse example of *Slums on the Drawing Boards* than Noble Street in Newcastle to which Benwell CDP (1976) applied that term. At least Noble Street was cheap rubbish. St Cuthberts was expensive rubblish.

Dunleavy (1981) concludes of this period that :

> Overall, families rehoused by urban authorities
> in the 1950s and 1960s probably received worse
> forms of accommodation than those rehoused in
> some earlier periods, despite improvements in
> design standards, heating and domestic equipment.
> The sharp alteration in the type of housing
> provided by public authorities coincided with
> a more gradual decline in the amenity of
> private housing developments at the lower end
> of the suburban market. But..both these trends
> took place in a period of rising standards of
> living in most other areas of social life. (p. 2)

Gateshead is an excellent illustration of this process.

CONCLUSION

In the introduction to this chapter three themes were identified, viz., 1) the understanding of the relationship between
housing and health outcomes - the social epidemiology of
housing and health ; 2) the contribution of this understanding to the formation of housing policy ; 3) the health consequences of housing policies themselves. In considering these
themes, what is remarkable, is the way in which in the late
1950s the 'health' dimension of housing was, to all intents
and purposes, forgotten. From the point of view of the state,
housing policy was the product of health requirements in the
nineteenth century. Although in the twentieth century 'class
action' in terms of demands for high quality provision assumed great importance, until the 1950s this was itself in part
a derivative of a concern with health. Clearly, it owed much
of its origins to the fact that state intervention in housing
for health reasons made housing part of the political process.

Why did the health dimension disappear? One possible explanation lies in the nature of the housing stock in the late
1950s and the early 1960s. By that time almost all the tenements of the early phase of industrial urbanisation had been
removed by slum clearance or bombing. The oldest housing
remaining was the first by-law housing of the 1860s. Much of
this was dilapidated but, given the regulation of its initial
quality, it was not usually sanitarily inadequate. Indeed,
by the mid 1960s clearance schemes were frequently resisted

by residents who took the greatest exception to having their
dwellings described as slums. Dennis (1970) documented this
process in detail for the Millfield area of Sunderland. He
identifies the change in the character of stock very precise-
ly :

> In contrast to the view of the MHLG's Development
> Group's Principal Architect that three million
> dwellings ought to be demolished, one of his
> colleagues at the Ministry believes that 'probably
> no other country possesses so large an inheritance
> of basically sound older houses'.(p. 20)

Dennis quotes this colleague :

> While in the past many of the houses we have
> been clearing have been obvious slums by any
> standards, rotten, damp, ruinous, verminous,
> the houses towards which health inspectors are
> now beginning to turn their attention are
> increasingly of a much better kind, and although
> in one or more respects they may be sub-standard
> it is often a simple matter to put them right.
> (Colin Jones, 1967, p. 4)

Dennis' work, and a review of other clearance schemes of
this period, makes it clear that by the mid 1960s it was not
generally possible to use 'health' as grounds for clearance
and that dilapidation, age, competition for site use, and
planners' prejuidices had replaced the clear social epidemiology of housing and health of the 1930s. Given the absence
of a health justification for clearance, the lack of attention to health factors in the design of the replacement stock
is easier to understand. In the 1930s people who were 'slum
cleared' did get much 'healthier' housing. The impact of the
change on their health was complicated given the impact of
higher rent levels on diet but there was no disagreement about
the improvement in the housing. By the middle of the 1960s
there was already extensive popular disquiet about 'mass
housing'. A lot of ordinary people were denying that the
'new housing' was better housing and in this they were well
ahead of the relevant professionals. The design departures
of the 1960s abandoned the health content of earlier forms.
The slum clearance replacement housing of the 1930s was less
good than the 'homes fit for heroes' of 1919 but it was often
recognisably the same sort of thing. It can often be converted into top quality stock, as was done on the Meadowell
Estate in North Shields in the middle 1970s when pairs of
flats were converted with considerable success into terraced

houses. If a house is a machine for living, 1930s stock might be regarded as two cylinder instead of six, but at least it worked. The mass housing of the 1950s to 70s was a 'departure in principle' and will be referred to again, but the hard won experience of a hundred years was dropped for a complex of reasons in which the profit of large construction companies loomed very large indeed. This is where the third theme resurfaces. By the mid 1970s problems of housing and health were, according to Fox and Goldblatt (1978), problems of council housing. The historical review set out above explains why this was so. The 'unhealthy housing' of earlier industrial urbanisation was very largely gone. The biggest contribution to contemporary 'unhealthy housing' was likely to be made by houses for the poor, designed and constructed without much reference to health. By the 1970s this was being recognised and that recognition is the subject matter of the next chapter of this book.

2 The contemporary situation

As has been noted in Chapter 1, the wealth of research and associated policy responses in the field of housing and health became a mere trickle by the 1950s and 1960s. It was widely felt that the backbone of the problem had been broken and that the knowledge and resources were available to tackle effectively the residue of bad housing and its associated effects on the health of the occupants.

Chapter 1 made extensive use of local Gateshead material. As was pointed out, there are already some excellent accounts available of the national scene, to which the reader can refer. In addition, much of the research, carried out as it was by practitioner researchers, was local in orientation. This chapter, however, takes a rather different approach. The 'trickle' of research on housing and health nationally in recent years was reflected in a similar 'trickle' at the local level in Gateshead. This chapter will thus of necessity cast its net wider, to glean what information and ideas are available. It will examine the challenge to the relative complacency of the 1950s and 1960s. These challenges, as will be seen, emerged both from criticisms of the accuracy and of the nature of this information: how far it was relevant to contemporary housing needs and how far it conveyed the effects on health of housing form and conditions.

Chapter 1 demonstrated the dramatic improvements in the housing conditions of the population over the twentieth century, as measured along a number of dimensions relating to structural condition, possession of 'basic' amenities and density of occupation. The last two types of indicators have been particularly popular and paint a particularly optimistic picture. Thus, by 1982, General Household Survey (GHS) data suggest that a very small proportion of households are badly housed according to these criteria. Ninety seven per cent in Great Britain had sole use of a bath or shower and 96 per cent sole use of an inside toilet. Fewer than one per cent lived at densities of more than one and a half persons per room and five per cent had one or more bedrooms fewer than the GHS standard (OPCS 1984, Tables 5.2, 5.3 and 5.25).

Poor housing by these criteria is not of course equally distributed among the population, between social classes, between regions or between tenures. The considerable variability in the housing circumstances of the population mean that average figures are in a very important, although not statistical sense, inaccurate. 'Pockets' of accommodation which are very deprived can still be found, most evidently in some inner city areas. In 1979-1980, for example, in the Inner London Borough of Hackney, 20 per cent of the dwellings were unfit for human habitation and a further 22 per cent in substantial disrepair (Harrison, 1983). However, the fact that these can be described as 'pockets' and contrasted so starkly with conditions achieved by the majority, reinforces the notion that improvements have been dramatic and that what remains is a residual, if particularly intractable, problem.

Townsend (1979) argues that some of the information behind this optimistic picture, especially that relying on local authority returns and forecasts, has tended to underestimate the scale and severity of housing problems. He refers to the unsubstantiated claims of successive politicians that the back of the 'slum problem' would be broken within a few years. He quotes the example of a survey carried out by public health inspectors in the mid 1960s, which found 1.8 million unfit dwellings in England and Wales, compared with local authority estimates of 820,000.

More recently, official studies have led to concern over the apparent failure of housing policies to provide further overall improvement in the structural condition of the housing stock. Unfit and structurally unsound housing is being replaced or demolished, but other houses are declining into an unsatisfactory condition at an even faster rate. Thus, the number of unfit dwellings in England has not been substantially reduced since 1971 and the situation in London and the South East has deteriorated. The number of dwellings needing substantial repairs increased by 22 per cent between 1976 and 1981 (Department of the Environment, 1982).

The acceptable minimum level of these traditional indicators of housing quality have been defined in a series of Public Health Acts as well as Housing Acts and a variety of government surveys. In other words, their relationship to health has been explicitly acknowledged. They have not remained immutable: for example, from 1961, the official census definition of overcrowding was reduced from two or more to more than one and a half persons per room (OPCS, 1963). However, the statutory definition has remained at the former level - as laid down in the 1935 Housing Act. As Ormandy (1981) points out, this means that the average two storeyed, terraced house (with three bedrooms, a living room and a kitchen) could be occupied by six adults and eight children aged between one year and ten years and still not defined as overcrowded.

Yet another 'official' definition of overcrowding has been adopted in recent years by the General Household Survey - published annually. Instead of counting all rooms except small kitchens, bathrooms and toilets as available for sleeping accommodation, this only includes bedrooms. Dwellings are defined as being overcrowded according to this 'bedroom standard' if any two people over the age of 21 (except a married couple) or any two people of different sexes aged 10 - 20, or more than two children under the age of 10 have to share a bedroom. The 1982 GHS found five per cent of households one or more bedrooms below this standard (OPCS, 1984, Table 5.25).

Part of the rationale for the development of a public sector in housing was of course the improvement of the quality of housing, especially that available to the working class. Local authority housing scores well relative to other tenures on many of the traditional indicators, although not as well on density of occupation (OPCS, 1984, Tables 5.19, 5.24, 5.25). In addition, unlike private sector dwellings, much building in the public sector has followed the space standards laid down by a series of government committes. The most recent and most generous standards were those recommended in 1961, by the Parker Morris Committee (MHLG, 1961), although since 1981 local authorities no longer have to build according to these standards to qualify for central government subsidies.

It may come, then, as something of a surprise to anyone with no familiarity with the council housing stock in Britain to read comments such as those of Townsend (1979):

> Our analysis suggests that, with the decline of
> privately rented housing, council housing is beginning
> to take its place as the sector with the largest
> number of deprived houses. (p.495)

In order to understand this type of argument, it is necessary
to consider the challenges of Townsend and others to traditional indicators of housing quality and the generally optimistic picture they convey. Firstly, there is the question of
how far they reflect minimum standards which are of contemporary relevance. As housing standards generally have risen,
dwellings which fall below these minima (and those which just
achieve them) provide housing which falls further and further
behind not only the standards achieved by the more privileged
households, but also those achieved by the great majority.
One way of interpreting this trend is to see it as a measure
of success in substantially reducing the incidence of housing
deprivation. Another way, however, is to argue that the minima
themselves should be raised to take account of changes in the
overall distributional framework of housing. These two inter-
pretations derive from rather different notions of deprivation.
The former suggests that we compare the housing circumstances
of people with some 'objective' and (theoretically) unchanging
notion of the minima necessary to sustain health and decency.
The latter suggests that the housing circumstances of people
should rather be compared with those of other people living at
the same time, in the same society. The former tends towards
an absolute, the latter towards a relative concept of deprivation (Townsend, 1979).

Thus, with regard to possession of 'basic' amenities,
Townsend (1979) suggests that, ideally, all household facilities should be listed, including telephones, central heating,
number of rooms normally heated in winter, waste disposal units
and double glazed windows, an adequate number of electrical
points and possession of consumer durables such as washing
machines, refrigerators, freezers and dishwashers. Households
could then be located along a continuum of deprivation/privi-
lege and their position assessed relative to the median, the
mode or the most privileged. Townsend found that council
tenants fared relatively well in terms of traditional basic
facilities, but suggests that their position would look rather
different if a wider range was included.

Unacceptable densities of occupation could similarly be
related to the standards achieved by the majority of the population. Harrison (1983) in his description of housing conditions in Hackney cites a number of examples where families are
not considered by the local authority to be overcrowded,

yet are living in cramped conditions, often in council accommodation, which appear to the reader and to the families themselves to be clearly unacceptable. Townsend (1979) found the
proportion of council tenants with insufficient bedrooms to be
about the same as those in the private rented sector and more
than those who were owner occupiers.

It has already been noted that the incidence of structural
defects so severe as to render the dwelling unfit for human
habitation is likely to be underestimated by local authority
returns. Less obvious and severe defects are even less likely
to come to the attention of the authorities, although the
English House Condition Survey provides periodic information
based on a sample of dwellings (DoE, 1978, 1982). Townsend
(1979) asked people in his survey if their housing had structural defects and about twice the proportion of council tenants
(27 per cent) as of owner occupiers responded that they had.
Only those living in privately rented unfurnished accommodation
reported more defects.

In the case of dampness, one of the major traditional
structural defects, there have even been attempts to redefine
some forms of damp as 'condensation' and to argue that this
is not a structural defect, but a consequence of improper use
of ventilation and central heating systems by the occupants.
If this is so, it could be argued that the structural defect
lay in the original installation of inefficient and expensive
to run central heating systems.

'Damp' or 'condensation' problems of this nature are associated particularly with public sector housing. This sector has
also been faced with a high incidence of other structural
defects, not only, as one would expect, in the older stock of
housing, built fifty or more years ago, but also in newer
housing. It is not so much that building for the private
sector has been of a particularly high quality, but that the
houses have tended to be of a more traditional nature and
involve more tried and tested methods of construction. It
could be argued that this is partly due to the private sect-
or's awareness of what prospective housebuyers want. In the
public sector, however, there has been more opportunity for
architects to realise their sculptural dreams, for local
authorities to enact their visions of the future and for large
building firms to propagate new building methods, produce
economies of scale and strengthen their market position.

The most striking example of these inter-tenurial differences
has been the substantial number of multi-dwelling units, or
flats, built for council tenants compared with their very minor

role in the owner occupied sector.

In 1977, over 30 per cent of council tenants lived in flats compared to around five per cent of owner occupiers (DoE, 1979b Table 2). Much of this 'mass housing' as Dunleavy calls it (1981) was built using new and untried methods. The amount of building meant that mistakes, when made, were made on a large scale. A Family Service Unit discussion paper (1983) on the problems of council housing quotes a housing researcher as saying:

> ...the use of experimental building methods and
> materials....have been the major source of problems
> in the experimental high rise blocks....the long-
> term maintenance requirements or the long-term
> durability have never been tested or approved. (p. 16)

Later in the same publication, a tenant comments:

> Our flats won't last another ten years, they are
> rotten now on the outside. They are terrible,
> they've only been up nine years. Bad workmen,
> shoddy workmanship, bad materials. (p. 32)

Townsend found in his 1969 survey that 22 per cent of the tenants of council dwellings built after 1955 reported struct-ural defects and he attributed this partly to the trend to-wards building flats rather than houses. Altogether he found that council tenants accounted for one-third of the population in property with structural defects.

However, the critique of public sector housing rests on more than performance on these traditional measures of structural defects. It rests also on a broader definition of housing quality, taking more aspects of that quality into account. For example, it has increasingly been argued that the location and environment of dwellings are important dimensions of hous-ing conditions:

> A house which offers everything a man or woman
> could desire when considered as a building may
> be uninhabitable when considered as a location.
> (Donnison and Ungerson, 1982, p. 12)

> What is required is a concept of 'environmental
> poverty' which includes the lack of or difficulty
> of access to gardens, play spaces, parks, water,
> shopping facilities and health centres, and takes
> account of exposure to noise and dirt. (Townsend, 1973)

Most of the households living in flats do not have access to
a garden or private outdoor play space, even though many were
originally built for families with children. Many public
sector dwellings are on estates which lack community provision
such as shops, health centres, social and recreational
facilities for adults, young people and children. Unreliable
or expensive public transport may make access to more distant
facilities difficult for many people. Donnison and Ungerson
(1982) suggest one reason why these environmental features
were so strikingly neglected in much public provision:

> Anyone who saw the overcrowding and squalor suffered
> until recently by people on the waiting lists in
> some of Britain's biggest cities must have some
> sympathy with elected representatives who demanded above
> everything else that more houses be built.
> To add a community centre, a bar or some shops
> to an estate might mean that families would have
> to wait longer in intolerable conditions.
> (pp. 254-255)

In recent years, some studies have attempted to measure the
quality of the environment. For example, the National Dwelling
and Housing Survey (DoE, 1979b) asked respondents about satisfaction not just with their accommodation, but with the area
in which they lived. While 8.7 per cent expressed dissatisfaction with their accommodation, 12.2 per cent were dissatisfied with the area. There were marked differences between the
tenures, with owner occupiers, as one would expect, least
dissatisfied. However, the differences were far less in relation to the area than they were in relation to the accommodation itself, maybe because the differences in the extent to
which the occupants can mould their accommodation to their own
requirements are greater than those with regard to shaping the
environment.

Townsend, in his 1969 poverty survey (1979), concentrated on
three measures of quality of housing environment: size of garden (if any); safe outdoor playing spaces for families with
children; and air pollution. He found that the three were highly correlated, with more than one quarter of households deprived on the first and third measures and about one-third of children deprived on the second. However, with the exception of
sole access to a garden, council tenants emerged as no more
deprived than owner occupiers, the other main tenure for
families with children.

This emphasises the point that not all council housing
suffers from defects and problems such as those discussed

above. There is considerable heterogeneity in this, as in other tenures. Much council housing is well built, well maintained and provides accommodation with which the occupants are quite content. Levels of expressed dissatisfaction are higher overall than in the owner occupied sector, although this may be partly the result of owner occupiers being less prepared to voice dissatisfaction about a property which they themselves have bought and maintained. Dissatisfaction is also more widespread among the occupants of flats and maisonettes as opposed to houses, which may account for some of the differences between tenures. However, many council tenants express a high degree of satisfaction (DoE, 1979b, Table 13).

Poor council housing is particularly associated with what have become known as 'difficult to let' estates. Many of these estates were built after the second world war. A postal survey in 1974 found that just under one-third of local authorities reported having at least one 'difficult to let' estate built since 1945. Over half of these had been built since 1965 (nine years or less before the survey) and two-thirds were in the form of flats and maisonettes (Taylor 1979). Often built with high hopes, if not high quality materials, for a variety of reasons, these estates have experienced a downward spiral in their state and status. The dwellings themselves have deteriorated and the environment has become increasingly barren and deprived physically and socially. As the estates have acquired an undesirable reputation, so no-one except the most desperate has been prepared to accept tenancies. Thus deprivation is intensified, with a concentration of households with social and economic difficulties (Harrison, 1983). As Taylor points out, to call these estates 'difficult to let' is to define the problem from a managerial perspective. For the tenants, they are most appropriately described as 'difficult to live in' and, in many cases 'difficult to get out of' (Taylor 1979). Local authorities have resorted in some of the most extreme cases to demolition and, more recently, to attempts to sell off properties to private commercial companies or to tenants' cooperatives. However, many still remain and, as the sale of the better council stock proceeds, they come to occupy a more and more significant role in the public sector.

However, what has all this to do with health? Is it valid to argue that these new forms of housing deprivation are associated with health consequences in the same way as over-crowding was linked with tuberculosis? The Black Report (DHSS, 1980) did report some evidence of greater mortality in the public sector. Standardising for occupational class, mortality rates for males aged 15-64 years were higher for council tenants than either owner occupiers or private tenants.

Mortality rates are often considered to be the most reliable indicators of ill health, but do not enable an assessment of overall morbidity. In addition, factors other than the nature of the housing itself may well be of importance. The health of an individual is influenced by a whole range of factors, of which housing is only one. Many of these, such as income, consumption habits, life style and working environment, as well as housing, are linked with social class and it is very difficult to disentangle the independent effects of any single factor. To complicate the picture further, council housing is unique in being the only tenure to which access can be gained through demonstrating medical need for a better stand- ard (or different type) of housing. Even though a relatively small proportion of council tenancies are granted on this 'medical priority' basis, this, together with the rehousing of individuals occupying some of the poorer quality private stock introduces some doubt as to the direction of the relationship for council tenants between their housing and their health. The point has even been made that improved housing may result in poorer health if the improvements result in higher housing and related costs, which mean individuals and families have less to spend on items equally important for health, particul- arly food (Donnison and Ungerson, 1982).

However, several studies have suggested that new forms of housing deprivation do have injurious effects on health and that these are particularly associated with 'mass housing' in the public sector. Most attention has been directed towards symptoms of respiratory disease (traditionally linked with bad housing) and symptoms of mental illness, particularly of the depressive type (an area of ill health not discussed so widely in earlier research). Far more attention has been paid than in the past to the opinions of those who actually live in the houses, as well as the 'experts' who are most likely to be aware of their ill health: the general practitio- ners. Small scale and exploratory studies have also tended to replace larger scale research into ecological variations.

Flats, including high rise flats, have attracted the great- est attention and this has been particularly directed towards the influence of living above ground level on the health of mothers and young children. Most are housed in the public sector, which accommodates something over one-third of all children, but well over three-quarters of those living above the first floor (Littlewood and Tinker, 1981). Hird (1966), in one of the first studies, found a substantial increase in the incidence of respiratory infections among children and in the number of consultations involving 'emotional disturbance'

among flat dwellers compared with house dwellers. Soon after,
Fanning (1967) published an article in the *British Medical
Journal* which has since frequently been cited and discussed in
which the morbidity of two groups of families of servicemen in
Germany, one group living in houses and the other in flats
was compared. He points to the similarities in design and
layout between these army quarters and modern English local
authority estates. The houses and the flats were of comparable age and quality of construction. He found, using a
number of indicators that:

> ... the morbidity of families living in flats was
> 57% higher than of those living in houses and that
> the greatest differences were seen in the incidence
> of respiratory infections in young women and children
> and of psycho-neurotic disorders in women. (p. 386)

Moreover the incidence of psychoneurosis increased with the
height of the residence in the blocks of flats, being twice
as high for those living on the top (third) floor as for those
living on the ground floor. Fanning goes on:

> The reasons for the differences in respiratory
> infections were felt to be the relatively small
> space available in a flat compared with that in
> a house, and confinement of the family within
> the flat. This confinement, and the resulting
> social isolation, were thought to be the reasons
> for the increase in psycho-neuroses in the women.
> (p. 386)

Gittus' study of, *Flats, Families and the Under Fives* (1976)
highlighted another potential danger to health of living off
ground level. This study is of particular interest as the
fieldwork was carried out in three Tyneside areas, one of
which was Gateshead. The focus was on mothers with preschool
children living in high rise blocks. Many of the mothers
interviewed mentioned spontaneously their concern about the
risk of accidents to their children who could fall from the
balconies or windows of the flats or be injured on the stairs
and fire escapes or in the lifts. These dangers were brought
home horrifically to the residents and to the survey team
when, during the fieldwork period, two young children were
killed in separate falls from windows in the blocks surveyed.

In addition, between one-half and two-thirds of the mothers
in the flats felt that they were adversely affected by living
in their present home, particularly that they felt more 'nervy'
and irritable. They reported adverse affects on between one-

quarter and one-half of their children under five chiefly associated with their isolation and restrictions on outdoor play.

More recently, Littlewood and Tinker's study for the Department of the Environment (1981) confirmed these findings. Almost two-thirds of the mothers they interviewed living off the ground floor regarded their accommodation as unsafe for children. The most anxious were those with two to four year old children and they were particularly worried about the stairs, balconies and windows. The authors estimated that a child was 57 times more likely to be killed if the home was above the first floor than if it was on the ground or first floors, although this risk, for all children is very small. The anxiety it causes for parents and the restriction placed on children's activities may well, however, have more widespread effects on health. The research also confirmed that mothers of very young children, especially those living above the fourth floor, were more likely to experience nervous disorders.

These studies concentrate on the effects on morbidity of a certain form of housing (flats); one which is most commonly found in the public sector. Other studies have concentrated on the effects of the low quality of some of this housing, including much which has been built relatively recently. Bedale and Fletcher (1982) report on a pilot study in Manchester interviewing people living in council maisonettes built only twenty years before (in the early 1960s). The main complaints of tenants centred on the dampness, the cold (there was electric underfloor heating, but this was reported to be both expensive and inadequate), the noise and the dangers to children of falling from landings and stairs. They reported high levels of various symptoms of mental ill health and of respiratory infections in children and blamed these chiefly on their housing conditions. Many had not been to a doctor about their 'nerves' because they felt that he could do nothing while they had to remain in the same housing.

Brown and Harris's work (1978) in the late 1960s and early 1970s on the social origins of depression suggested that environmental difficulties are associated with a greater likelihood of depressive illness in women and that these explain much of the social class differences in incidence. Housing was found to be one of the most important of these difficulties. Of those women they interviewed who were defined as suffering from chronic psychiatric conditions, 28 per cent had a 'major housing difficulty', compared with only six per cent of those not suffering from such conditions. The authors argue that the housing difficulties probably contributed directly to the perpetuation of the psychiatric condition especially in the feelings of hopelessness and low self worth generated, leaving aside any role they might also have played in the original onset. However, they emphasise the problems in establishing a direct causal link:

> Poor housing is often linked with marital and
> other problems (in the aetiology of psychiatric
> conditions) in a way that makes interpretation
> of causal processes hazardous. (pp. 199-200)

Much of the evidence that housing, which would often not by traditional measures be considered as substandard, has damaging effects on health is open to challenge. Correlation does not necessarily imply a causal relationship, even where, as in Bedale's study the respondents themselves make the link.

Littlewood and Tinker (1981) reported that, contrary to popular assumptions, their survey could find no evidence that living in flats at any level had a detrimental effect on child development if children of similar backgrounds are compared. However, the degree of marital satisfaction with the family's housing did have an effect and so, as more mothers living above first floor level were likely to be dissatisfied, then children living at these levels as a group performed less well at school and demonstrated more disturbed behaviour.

Even where housing conditions are evidently bad, there is often no clear evidence that they produce ill health. For example, a 1981 article in *Roof*, (Franey, 1981) quotes a specialist in community medicine as saying:

> One tends to assume that bad health and bad
> housing go together, but in reality it's very
> difficult to prove. You see, a tenant's ill
> health could be due to a hundred things...With
> damp there is no evidence that it causes bad health.
> One of our environmental health officers spent
> days in the library looking up all the medical
> studies and he couldn't find anything to link
> the two. (p. 11)

Muir Grey (1978), an Oxford community physician and medical adviser to the local housing committee, analysed 612 of the applications he had received for medical priority in the allocation of council housing. He was unable to find a single case where the housing conditions definitely caused physical (or mental) disease.

One recent study which cast considerable doubts on the
existence of a causal relationship was that of Pike and his
colleagues (1981), who looked at morbidity and environment in
an urban general practice in Birmingham in the late 1970s.
They compared morbidity (measured by clinical activity with
respect to patients) in two different areas in which practice
patients lived and also considered changes over time in
morbidity in areas which had undergone considerable renovation
and improvement. They concluded that their investigations
were unable to demonstrate:

(a)   That living in an area of deprivation leads
      to more episodes of illness,

(b)   That renovating old houses and improving the
      external appearance of housing and their
      surroundings leads to less episodes of illness.
      (p. 71)

Bedale and Fletcher (1982) have criticised these findings:
for example, the study made assumptions about the housing
conditions of a relatively small proportion of individuals
living in a particular area from census generated data about
differences between areas as a whole. It was also assumed
that housing in the inner city area was worse than that on
outer ring council estates. Although it may have appeared
worse on census indicators, as discussed above, these may not
be particularly accurate measures of overall quality. Improvement policies only began near to the end of the research
period and had not produced substantial benefits, thus it is
not surprising that little improvement in health was evident.
Measurements of health relied on indicators of the use of
medical services which the authors, Pike et al (1981), recognise
as inadequate. They suggest further research using broader
measures of health, including subjective measures collected,
for example, by the completion of health diaries by respondents.

The importance of subjective measures is emphasised by
Tudor Hart, a physician who is well known as the formulator of
the 'inverse care law', whereby the quantity and quality of
medical services available is inversely related to the level
of need. He argued:

It is a serious mistake to get drawn into pseudo-
scientific arguments about whether there is a
causal association between bad health and poor
housing...a link between respiratory disease and
damp homes is neither proved nor provable because
you can't isolate it from all the other factors

43

that are inevitably associated with the two...
Yet in 30 years of practice...I have never seen
rehousing into a decent place have anything but
a good effect on a family's health...Bad housing
wears down self esteem...it undermines physical
health. We don't need to prove medically that
dampness causes disease - it is enough that it
makes us feel rotten. (Quoted in Franey, 1981,
pp. 11-12)

It is perhaps useful here to distinguish between housing of
such a low quality, poor design and so badly located that it
would be likely to have damaging health consequences for any
occupant, and housing which is only harmful to the health of
particular types of individuals or families because of their
physical, social or health characteristics. Flats are a good
example of this. Some developments such as those described by
Harrison (1983), are very difficult to let, unpopular with
almost everyone who lives there, many of whom will be trying
to get out, and are found to have severe design and structural
faults. Others, however, have been particularly criticised
for their unsuitability for particular types of tenant.
Families with young children are the best known example, but
the chronically ill may find stairs a problem and isolation
a source of anxiety. Developments which, with all good
intentions, provide for a mix of different types and ages of
households, can pose problems because of conflicts of interests and lifestyles, especially where there are high densities
of children and young people.

These latter types of problems can, to some degree at least,
be overcome by alterations in allocation policies and opportunities for transfer. Thus, for example, many local authorities (Gateshead is one) now have a policy of not allocating
families with young children to dwellings on the upper floors
of high rise accommodation (Littlewood and Tinker, 1981). The
'medical priority' system of allocating council houses includes categories for granting new tenancies to individuals who
have developed an illness which makes previously satisfactory
accommodation unsuitable (Muir Grey, 1978). How far this
'reshuffling' is possible depends of course on the mix of
local authority tenants and potential tenants and the variety
of housing available. As council house sales reduce not just
the quantity, but also the quality and variety of the stock
(given that higher quality dwellings of a particular form -
houses rather than flats - are more likely to be sold), it is
probable that local housing committees will have less scope
to offer appropriate accommodation to various categories of
tenants.

However, difficult as this exercise may be, the problems associated with poor quality,'difficult to let' housing can necessitate far more drastic action. Local authorities can face massive bills for major repairs and renovation. In some cases the decision has been taken actually to demolish the housing, well before the loans taken out to build it have been repaid (DoE, 1980 c). In addition to the continuing repayments of these loan charges and the costs of demolition, the local authority may well be faced with extra expenditure associated with finding accommodation for displaced tenants.

3 Conceptualising and carrying out the study

INTRODUCTION

The historical and contemporary accounts of the relationships between housing and health lead in this chapter to a consideration of the nature of further investigations of these relationships in the 'housing and health' study. The chapter divides into two sections. In the first, broad methodological issues relating to explanation and investigation of housing, health and class are discussed. The second consists of an account of how the study was carried out: the sampling of housing areas and households, the structure of the interviews, the conduct of the survey and the subsequent analyses of data. Both of these sections are of central importance to the study as a whole, as one important element in the original research plans was to investigate ways of doing research in this field.

CONCEPTUALISING THE STUDY

In a recent article Blume (1982) has asserted that three distinctive intellectual traditions can be identified in investigations of inequalities in rates of sickness and mortality among social groups: social administration, epidemiology and sociology. These, he argues, differ with regard to, "... how 'the problem' is conceptualized" (p. 8).

In summary description:

> ...social administration focuses upon unequal
> provision of services, and upon factors leading
> to lower utilization by the working classes in
> relation to their needs. Its interest in disease(s)
> is on the whole limited by the extent to which
> demonstrable relationships with the results of
> collective provision and material circumstances
> are to be found. Epidemiology is concerned to
> explore the aetiology of specific diseases,
> implicating specific social conditions and aspects
> of the physical environment, especially in so far
> as medically plausible intervening factors can
> be postulated. Sociology, like social administration,
> is on safest ground in dealing with the structure
> of health services. Unlike social administration,
> however, its explanation of these structures
> (including those aspects leading to under-utilization
> by low status or working class groups) is in terms
> of theoretically grounded variables generally
> employed within sociology for explaining social
> structure and processes. Liberation of concepts
> of health/disease from medical diagnostic categories
> - health as well-being - broadens the field within
> which sociology seems applicable. (pp. 24-25)

However, although Blume's article is very useful in prompting the articulation of important issues, it can be argued
that he fails to develop these issues. Three can be identified here:

1)   Aggregate explanation versus individual explanation.

2)   The nature of appropriate intervention.

3)   'Adequacy at the level of meaning'.

Blume (1982) in his discussion of frames of reference in
epidemiology says:

> My argument is that the kind of linkages which
> epidemiologists seek are those which are plausible
> from, legitimated by, a clinical medical perspective...
> Epidemiology is at root no less individualistic
> than are the basic biomedical sciences with which
> it is linked in a common endeavour. (p. 18, p.26)

These statements describe accurately the contemporary nature
of epidemiology, but are completely at variance with the

nature of epidemiology in recent history, and in particular
with the 'social epidemiology of housing and health'. For
example, in his account of the causes of tuberculosis,
Bradbury (1933) was perfectly clear about the 'biomedical
scientific' explanation in individualistic terms. Tuberculosis was caused by the tubercule bacillus. What interested
him were the factors which predisposed towards 'infection or
proliferation'. So far his approach was very close to that
which Blume endorses, that is, Brown and Harris's model (1978)
which posits:

> ...two essential but quite distinct kinds of
> variables in interaction: first what might be
> called the structural-environmental factors, and
> second 'host' factors, or what Brown and Harris term
> vulnerability factors. The first includes all
> aspects of the social structure, of the social
> and physical environment with potential implications
> for health and disease... The second set of factors
> includes all those characteristics of the individual
> which might singly or in interaction affect his
> or her susceptibility to disease. (pp. 27-28)

Bradbury collected information about cases but his focus of
analysis was on aggregates, on collectivities, and his prescriptions were collective rather than individualistic. This
distinction is very important. Blume, who provided structure
for this argument, interprets Brown and Harris's important
work in individualistic terms at the level of prescription -
the level of prescription of contemporary clinical medicine
and the level of explanation of biomedical science. Classical
epidemiology was not so constructed. Navarro (1978) has
argued that the status of contemporary curative medicine is
parasitic on the achievements of social and preventive
medicine in every sense. This argument has much force,
especially in relation to collective prevention.

Blume places considerable emphasis on contemporary epidemiology's concern with consumption habits. Such habits, while
socially and culturally generated, insofar as they are held to
be functions of individual choice rather than collective
restraint, are dealt with by individual prescription. They
can be assimilated into the practice of clinical medicine.
General structural factors, such as the prevalence of asbestos
in work places and in much mass housing, cannot be prescribed
for at this individual level. They require collective action
in a political context. This is the focus of the second
category of issues: the nature of appropriate intervention.
Social administration, which for the authors is the study of,
and elaboration of, policies, has always emphasised the

collective, although it has not always employed the categories of class.

The third issue is about 'adequacy at the level of meaning'. Catherine Marsh (1982) in a book which is important in its relation to the whole of the research process here described, has written:

> The aim of explanation is not just to show high correlations...It must also show how the actions of the people involved were the actions of conscious human beings, reacting to an environment, trying to make sense of it, and pursuing various goals in their actions with more or less success. Only explanations which take cognisance of the meaningful aspect of social action will satisfy us as human observers. (p. 98)

Marsh clearly identifies the division within sociology between those approaches which emphasise structure and those which emphasis social meaning. It is perfectly possible to generate collectively orientated, structurally located explanations, with a model of political action as approriate intervention, which completely leaves out people as subjective actors with consciousnesses. As Avineri (1966) points out, this is the epistemological position shared by crude Leninism and right wing social democracy.

The above discussion leads, if in a somewhat roundabout way, to the central aim of this section: the specification of the components of a model of exploration and investigation (and the apparent reverse ordering of those words is quite deliberate) which is socio-historically adequate. In other words, a model which makes sense in relation to the historical account which constitutes the first chapter of this book. It is not the elaboration of the model, or explanatory framework, which is particularly difficult but rather how that model can be translated into an investigation of the real world.

Firstly, the specification of components of the model requires collecting information from subjects who are aware of the nature of and the meanings they attach to this information. It has to be of such a character that it can be historically located in relation to a social epidemiology which explores differences between collectivities (for example, social classes). Questions then arise of how this information is to be collected and how it can be analysed and utilised.

Collecting 'real' knowledge - the survey process

This book and the research project on which it is based are about 'health', 'housing' and 'other relevant factors'. To talk about them in terms of a model it is necessary to specify first the general understanding of the social processes which are being modelled and then the relationship of the theoretical model to the real world through an operational definition. The problem of operationalisation consists of more than the measurement instructions involved in translating an element in a model, like health, into a set of measurement operations. Rather, the fundamental problem is how to access the world in order to measure. Raymond Williams (1982) has commented that the development of statistics in the 1840s was itself a product of industrial urbanisation: the significant world became too complex to know through direct personal observation. Quantification was a procedure for summarising the complexity. The social survey is the method which has been developed as a procedure for obtaining information for specific purposes. The use of this method has provoked a major methodological debate which it is not proposed to discuss here. As Marsh (1982) argues:

> Surveys have a lot to offer the sociologist.
> Since experimentation cannot be used to investigate
> a wide range of macro-social processes, there
> is often no alternative to considering variation
> across cases in a systematic fashion. Since the
> processes of determination in the social world
> are subjective in important ways, involving actors'
> meanings and intentions, the survey researcher has
> to face the task of measuring these subjective
> aspects. It is not easy. (p. 147)

Nonetheless, as Marsh implies, there is no reasonable alternative. This summary contains two important elements. One relates to the exploration of variation through the systematic consideration of values for different cases and will be returned to in the discussion of analytical procedures. The other has to do with subjective meaning. Bateson (1984) has discussed this in relation to three forms of survey knowledge:

a) knowledge as information, held in the heads of the informants and organised in the natural language of everyday life;

b) knowledge as data, constructed by the researcher using the standard measurement operations of the survey method and organised in the form of a classification scheme;

c) knowledge as expertise, held in the head of the survey client and organised in the form of summary values on variables and relationships among variables.

As was the case with Blume, Bateson's position is very useful as a point of departure; for him, the survey process is one of collecting information through the construction of 'data' for analysis in relation to expertise. However, the question of subjectivity remains.

In considering 'health', Doyal (1979) has reviewed the nature of definitions. She locates prevailing definitions of 'health' in terms of the absence of 'clearly observable pathological abnormality of function' in the context of a mechanistic scientific medical model which itself is derived from:

> ...the atomised individualistic world view which accompanied the rise of the capitalist mode of production. (pp. 238-239)

Bradbury's definition (1933) was of exactly this kind, i.e. differentiation among families on the basis of the presence or absence of clinically observeable tuberculosis in at least one family member. However, using this framework is not necessarily the best way to proceed. In her review of available information on the condition of the health of the UK population, Doyal identified the findings of the GHS as:

> ...the least unsatisfactory estimate of the state of health of the population...because: ...respondents are themselves asked about their health. (p. 246)

In any definition of 'health' which attempts to take account of its holistic and subjective character, people have to be asked what they feel. This tends to lead to a breakdown between the categories of information and expertise as suggested by Bateson, although the expert remains the manipulator and analyst of the 'data'. In the 'housing and health' survey, respondents were asked what they thought, not just about their health and their housing, but also about the relationship between them. This was very important as it enabled respondents to play an active part in the collection of 'knowledge as data'.

Other material was designed to elicit that which the clinician would elicit through standard diagnostic procedures. Questions about respiratory functions, mobility and depression came from previously validated questionnaire items which

involved asking respondents about their symptoms. Analyses
based on this type of material have their uses, but in the
present survey, priority was given to subjective assessments
of the respondents themselves.

It is important to note that this assertion is to some
considerable degree post hoc. The survey method of information collection was originally chosen because no bank of material covering the topics of central interest was available
for secondary analysis, although, clearly, aspects of the
relationships among housing and health and other factors can
be explored through the use of medical records, analyses of
census data and death certificates (see Fox and Goldblatt,
1978). However, as the study progressed it became increasingly evident that the use of subjective accounts was the most
appropriate since what people think is ultimately of prime
importance.

Operationalising social processes

The operationalisation of health has been discussed above in
the context of the collection of information and 'data'
construction. The operationalisation of housing is discussed
in relation to the design of the sampling procedures. In this
section, 'class' will be discussed in the context of the
exploration of models. The historical account of housing and
health in Chapter 1 was an account of working class housing
and health; underpinning it was a concern with the development of housing and health policy as a way of coping with the
problem of the reproduction of 'labour power' in industrial
urban society. The process of differentiation in housing
within the working class was the basis of the development of
good working class housing provided through a market mechan-
ism under state regulation in the latter half of the nineteenth century.

It was argued that council housing in the twentieth century
maintained this differentiation, albeit that the autonomous
action of the working class around issues of living standards
in general and housing in particular, modified the simple
relationship between level of income and housing standards.
These rather complex statements can be reduced to some simple
propositions.

1)   The working class is not homogeneous but can be divided
(in one useful formulation of a general idea) into 'central'
and 'peripheral' workers (see Friedman, 1977). Very crudely,
'peripheral' workers and the 'reserve army' of labour or
'surplus population' (see Friend and Metcalf, 1981) will have

difficulty in achieving what is generally considered to be an adequate standard of living. In contrast, 'central' workers, through their collective exercise of power, will be able to achieve a better standard of living through their wages. State benefit systems will thus be crucial to the lives of the 'peripheral' workers and the 'reserve army' as a means of attaining a minimally adequate income. It should be noted that this is a dynamic situation and 'central' workers can become 'peripheral' especially in conditions of economic crisis, and vice versa.

2) Working class action in housing has, in part, reproduced this distinction, but it has also challenged it. Poor people thus usually live in worse housing, but sometimes they do not.

The aim in this study was to determine the mechanisms by which housing, class and health happen together. Payne and Payne (1979), in an attempt to articulate a Weberian frame-work 'to guide research into the effects of social policy' asserted that:

> It is through the mechanism of housing that the
> major life experiences, conventionally associated
> with occupational class, are determined; housing's
> relevance for stratification is not just as an index
> of achieved life chances, but as a means by which
> the inequalities of the occupational structure are
> transferred into the wider social structure. The
> closer the fit between occupation and housing the
> more sharply stratified are social inequalities.
> (p. 134)

Until 1972, the existence of differential rents in council housing, which were a function of the historic cost and present esteem of particular dwellings, and the absence of rent rebates on a general scale meant that labour market derived income inequalities were important in conditioning access to differ-ent types of stock. That is much less the case now, although as the cluster analyses show (see Chapter 4) there is still a high degree of social differentiation. It was decided to attempt to operationalise the segmentation within the working class in a way which, however crudely, reflected the reality of social organisation in Gateshead in the 1980s.

This immediately raised a serious, and not easily resolved, question about the nature and levels of the units of analysis and the relationships among the units belonging to different levels. The problem is the classic one of hierarchical data analysis - the relationship between individuals and house-holds. The simplest definition of a household is one which emphasises, as a first criterion, occupation of the same dwelling. Clearly, 'housing conditions' operate in relation to the aggregate household. In the same way 'housing area' might be considered to operate in relation to an aggregate estate population. However, 'health' is almost always thought of as an individual characteristic. Interestingly, Bradbury (1933) did not think in this way. He talked about 'tubercular families' that is families characterised by the presence of tuberculosis in one or more members, and he related household conditions to this. In general, the present study relates housing and household factors to individual statements (or in the case of children, 'mother figure' statements), about health. It would have been useful to have related case to case (i.e. individual to individual) and to construct aggregate measures of household health but this was not technically possible.

The problem of an approriate method of coping with class was not easy to resolve. Usually, in epidemiological studies, Registrar General's social class is used without qualification. The Black Report (DHSS, 1980) is, to a considerable degree, a series of tables of inequalities in mortality broken down by age, sex and Registrar General's social class. Nichols (1979) defines the key criterion which any operationalisation of class has to be capable of meeting:

> ...at the heart of the matter are questions about
> who is on what side in the dominant relations of
> exploitation, what the consequences of this are
> and what they can be made to be. (pp. 167-168)

Social statisticians usually deal with class as an attribute of individuals who are the cases in analyses. However, using Nichol's criterion it is possible to conclude with E.P. Thompson (1978):

> ...class is not this or that part of the machine
> but the way the machine works once it is set in
> motion..Class is a social and cultural formation
> (often finding institutional expression) which
> cannot be defined abstractly or in isolation,
> but only in terms of relationships with other
> classes; and ultimately, the definition can only
> be made in the medium of time - that is action and
> reaction, change and conflict...class itself is not
> a thing, it is a happening. (p. 85)

It is very difficult to cope with this in the framework of a social survey which is, of necessity, a snapshot, however much an attempt is made to collect material about processes (as Bradbury did in his efforts at chronological ordering). One course would be to extend the time scale but this is always difficult. Another way is to attempt, in the construction of the data, to create categories which have something to do with present day reality. The following cases illustrate this. For example - one household consists of a husband of forty five, a skilled fitter in full time employment, with a wife who is a clerical worker with the local authority and a daughter who is a nurse. Another household consists of a husband of forty-five, a skilled fitter who has been unemployed for two years, whose wife does not work and who has three children at school. These two instances are very far from being extreme cases of households which, if classified by Registrar General's criteria (i.e. according to the occupation of the head of the household) would belong to both the same social class and the same socio-economic group. Yet one household could have a per capita income of more than four times that of the other.

For council tenants there is an administrative process which categorises according to a criterion of net resources per person in the household. This is the process of determining eligibility for housing benefit. It was decided to use this to produce a classification of 'household class', categorised into households as follows: those receiving no housing benefit and paying full rent; those receiving some housing benefit and paying some rent; and those who paid no rent in consequence of level of receipt of housing benefit (all members of such a household might be unemployed). Other ways of dealing with the relationship between a household's location in the production system and its resources have been used but this classification is a useful, if rather crude, operationalisation of peripheralisation/centrality. Households not in receipt of unified housing benefit can reproduce their labour power out of their own resources. Those in receipt of full rent benefit and those in the intermediate category cannot, but the latter households are not totally dependent on state benefits for maintenance. It was felt that the 'household class' of a household covered the non housing aspects of class rather well.

This is similar to Bradbury's use of 'poverty level' in 1933, but it should be noted that he confined himself to families as cases whereas in this study 'housing' and 'household class' were both assigned to individuals. Thus cross level inference was used and individuals were assigned properties of the collectivity (the household) of which they were a part. This is regularly done elsewhere without explication. In many ways, it would have been preferable to have been able to analyse at one level - to relate some aggregate measure of household health to housing and household class, and ways of doing this are being explored in another context.

Exploring historically grounded models

> Exploratory data analysis seeks to construct and test models against data collected from the social world. The models are intended to account for theoretically significant patterns in the data. In order to assess the validity of a model, an analytic technique is used to generate the data which would have been obtained if the model did correctly represent the real world, and this data and the observed data are compared. The essence of the exploratory approach to analysis is that successive models are examined to find that which best fits the data. (Gilbert, 1982, p, 7)

The analytical procedures employed in the 'housing and health' study are located in an exploratory mode, that is to say, the aim is to look for patterns, but, as Gilbert suggests, the models proposed are grounded in a 'theory' of what reality might be like. In the present study this is taken further. The historical relationship between housing and health is known and the interest lies in investigating whether, in a new housing system, that relationship remains. This means that the simple, study based induction proposed by Gilbert in the above quotation is not followed. It is not sufficient to identify the model that 'best fits' the data, although this will always be reported. A prime objective is to look to see if the historically grounded model remains applicable today.

This is, perhaps, operating even farther beyond the conventional boundaries of hypothetico-deductive analysis. Hellevik (1984) has pointed out that log-linear models, the subject of Gilbert's book (1982), are basically tests of fit, although:

> Sometimes models in a log-linear analysis are specified on the basis of theoretical reasoning in reference to the characteristics of the subject of study. A causal model may also contain assumptions for which the statistical analysis will decide whether they were correct or not, when it has been made specific by assuming that one or more effects are positive, negative or absent. But in addition it will always contain assumptions of a substantive nature, which the statistical analysis in itself cannot test. These concern the time ordering of the variables and the relationship between variables included in the

model and those left outside. Since they cannot
be justified by the results of the statistical
analyses, but rather constitute the foundation on
which this analysis rests, the researcher is forced
to rely on theoretical arguments or substantive
references to convince his audience that the
assumptions are reasonable. (p. 188)

The causal modelling proposed by Hellevik is employed in
association with some log-linear analyses as illustration,
but even in other analyses which do not involve log-linear
analyses this is the logic of the approach used. The implications of this are quite considerable. It asserts the priority of historical accounts over statistical reasoning and
regards quantitative procedures simply as a useful set of
tools in the development of historical accounts, not to be
employed in a positivist fashion. The major problem in locat-
ing this position is not in distinguishing it from the kind of
individualistic positivism which increasingly dominates
epidemiology. Rather it is in justifying any form of quantitative reasoning against both ethnomethodologists who deny the
epistemological validity of such approaches and naive popu-
lists who argue that quantification is inherently reactionary
in political terms. The authors believe that the collection
of the information that ordinary people have in their heads
matters. As far as possible it should be analysed in their
terms, but that does not confine the analysis to literary
representations of edited highlights of interviews (although
this is no way denies the validity and indeed desirability of
ethnographic explorations in this field).

This is to say that quite complicated quantitative models
have some place in all this, contrary to Tudor Hart's assertion (1981), already referred to in Chapter 2:

It is a serious mistake to get drawn into pseudo-
scientific arguments about whether there is a causal
association between bad health and poor housing...
a link between respiratory disease and damp houses
is neither proveable because you can't isolate it from
all the other factors that are inherently associated
with the two...We don't need to prove medically that
dampness causes disease. (Quoted in Franey, 1981; pp 11-12)

However, to contend with individualistic accounts of the
aetiology of collective morbidity it is necessary to pursue
that proof. The virtual abandonment of socially located
epidemiology, and in particular of the social epidemiology of
housing and health, is an important factor in determining the

nature of contemporary housing provision for working class people. A collectively orientated, quantitatively based, scientific approach to these issues is possible and ought to be attempted. It has to be complemented by history, ethnography and personal experience, but it has a part to play in what might, somewhat pretentiously, be called the cultural politics of policy formation. In the 1930s the social epidemiology of tuberculosis was used as important supporting evidence in working class pressure for better housing. The social epidemiology of the health consequences of mass housing has a similar part to play today.

CARRYING OUT THE STUDY

Introduction

The previous chapters commented on the fact that, although there have been substantial improvements in housing conditions and a decline in the incidence of virulance of diseases most clearly associated with poor housing, there are indications that problems remain. It was noted that, in relation to public sector housing, where conditions are by many measures the best, the Black Report on inequalities in health (DHSS, 1980) reported that such housing was associated with the highest rates of mortality. Brown and Harris's work (1978) on the social origins of depression suggested that certain forms of housing may have deleterious effects on mental health and the English House Condition Survey 1981 (DoE, 1982) showed that the number of houses needing repairs has increased substantially in recent years.

It was from this perspective that the study of the relationship between health and housing conditions in Gateshead developed. In the words of the grant submission, the study aimed to:

> ...identify the housing, health and relevant
> other conditions of households located in a range
> of public sector dwellings in a North Eastern
> Metropolitan District and to provide an explanation
> of the impact of housing form (1) and conditions on
> health, taking other relevant factors into account.

This is not an easy area in which to do research. Ill health is associated with many factors, such as genetic predisposition, age, sex, occupation, income and consumption habits, some of which are likely to co-vary with housing conditions. To add to the complexity, the public sector is unique in that poor health is, in itself, a factor in gaining

access to housing. However, the proportion of new tenancies
or transfers granted on the basis of medical priority in the
local authority studied was found to be sufficiently small to
prevent this being a substantial problem except, as is suggested later, in relation to elderly tenants.

The research was thus designed as a pilot study to explore
ways of doing research in this field and also to suggest
relations between health and housing which merit further
consideration on a wider scale.

Procedure

Classification and selection of council housing areas

This stage of the research aimed to develop a classification
of all council housing areas (CHAs) in Gateshead which would
enable a range of different types of council housing to be
distinguished. It was carried out by means of a two stage
cluster analysis of data sets describing the areas. This
analysis had the following nine sub-stages.

1) *Construction of Census level data set*

Using Small Area Statistics, a data file was created for
Gateshead containing 91 variables from the 1981 Census (100
per cent data) for each of the 489 enumeration districts
(EDs) which were nether 'special', i.e. consisted of something other than a set of ordinary private households, or
'restricted', i.e. contained so few private households (less
than eight or less than 25 persons) that the data relating
to them was not made available by OPCS as a protection of
the confidentiality of census respondents.

From the 91 variables, SPSS (Statistical Package for the
Social Sciences) was used to generate 46 census indices; 43
of the indices were percentages and three, (total persons;
total persons resident in private households; total private
households) were the bases for the percentages.

2) *Selection of 'council' EDs*

One of the census derived indices constructed at sub-stage
1) gave a figure for each ED for the percentage of private
households renting their dwelling from the local authority.
All EDs in which 60 per cent or more households were council
tenants were selected. This produced 209 'council' EDs.
The figure of 60 per cent was chosen because it was felt
that this figure represented an unequivocal majority of the
stock. In fact, 90 per cent of all households in the

'council' EDs were council households and the selected EDs contained most of the council housing in the Borough. That which was omitted tended to include some of the best stock, located in areas where the 'right to buy' has proved a popular option.

The 209 'council' EDs contained approximately 31,415 council households out of approximately 36,690 such households present in the 489 'ordinary' EDs (i.e. 86 per cent).

3)   *Classification of 'council' EDs*

The 209 'council' EDs were classified on the basis of a cluster analysis using a set of variables drawn from the overall set, chosen as being of most value in classifying residential locales for the purpose of a housing and health study. They relate to demographic characteristics, economic activity, housing conditions and turnover, morbidity, level of affluence and location of single parent families and students. The classification employed began from a random allocation of cases of one to ten clusters and proceeded with fusion according to Ward's method (Everitt, 1974). The data was in the form of percentages and was left in this state without standardisation thereby preserving the significance of absolute differences. Five clusters were generated which demonstrated a high level of stability.

4)   *Identification of CHAs*

CHAs were constructed consisting of 'council' EDs in the same cluster which were geographically contiguous or any free standing 'council' ED. From this, 87 CHAs were identified.

5)   *Construction of CHA data set*

A data set was constructed for the 87 CHAs consisting of an extended census data set (including variables from the 10 per cent Census data which was now available and which enabled the generation of a further 24 indices), together with data from the local housing authority relating to allocations, turnovers, voids (i.e. empty dwellings) and house purchases. This gave a total of 102 variables of which 70 were census-derived and 32 came from the local housing authority.

The 87 CHAs constructed from the 209 'council' EDs contained 89,650 people at the time of the 1981 Census. Of these, 89,130 lived in 33,360 private households of which 31,415 were council tenant households.

6)   *Classification of CHAs*

The 87 CHAs were classified on the basis of a cluster analysis using the extended data set. The variables used related to demographic characteristics, economic activity,
morbidity, incidence of single parents, housing conditions,
affluence, social class, housing turnover, empty dwellings,
medical priority and council house purchases. Classification generated five clusters which corresponded closely to
those of individual EDs. A brief description of the five
CHA clusters is given following the outline of the nine
sub-stages.

7)   *Sampling of CHAs*

The 87 CHAs were subjected to a two-way classification
based on cluster membership and whether they contained
predominantly flats or houses. This produced a total of
10 cells, of which eight were occupied. A sample of one
CHA was drawn from each of these on a basis which weighted
the chance of selection of a CHA according to the number of
EDs which it comprised. The eight CHAs thus sampled and
listed below, provided the locale for the second stage of
study, the interview survey.

Cluster	CHA
1 (mainly flats)	St Cuthberts Non traditional estate built in the 1960s. Medium rise maison-ettes and some high rise flats. Classified by the local author-ity as 'difficult to let'.
1 (mainly houses)	Old Fold Traditional low rise, prewar estate. Classified as 'difficult to let'.
2 (mainly flats)	Nursery Lane High rise estate built in the 1960s. Classified as 'difficult to let'.
3 (mainly flats)	Allerdene High rise estate built in the 1970s with high density of elderly residents.
3 (mainly houses)	Meadow Lane Low rise accommodation built in

the 1960s, mainly housing but
some 2-storey flats. High
density of elderly residents.

4 (mainly flats)   Carlisle Court
                       Medium rise estate built in the
                       1960s.

4 (mainly houses)   Wrekenton
                       Traditional low rise estate.
                       Built in the 1950s

5 (mainly houses)   Beacon Lough
                       Modern low rise estate. Built
                       in the 1970s.

8) *The sampling of households*

From each of the CHAs a sample of 60 households was drawn
by address. The sampling frame employed was the current
electoral register modified by comparison with the local
authority records of void properties and also by inspection.
A listing of occupied addresses was thus obtained and the
resident household interviewed. In some instances the
addresses were still clearly unoccupied and the interviewers were instructed to ascertain this by checking with
neighbours and then to replace the unoccupied address with
the nearest 'above' or 'below' address as indicated by
flipping a coin. Systematic sampling was used with a
randomly selected starting point and with a sampling fract-
ion in each CHA constructed so as to give a sample of 60
households for each CHA. Thus, the sampling procedure can
be described as two-stage; at the first stage stratified,
randomly selected, and with variable sampling fractions;
at the second stage quasi-randomly selected by systematic
sampling and with variable sampling fractions. This is
clearly a considerable departure from straightforward
random sampling but given the fact that the sampling fractions, particularly at the second stage, were such as to
give samples which were comparatively large in relation to
small populations, it was considered that this did not pose
major problems from the point of view of establishing significance levels. However it should be emphasised that the
stratification and variable sampling fractions employed at
the first stage, and the variable sampling fractions employed at the second stage have the effect of making the
total sample obtained by the combination of all households
from all CHAs sampled unrepresentative of the overall
population of Gateshead council households. In particular,

households resident on 'difficult to let' estates were
systematically over-represented in the sample in comparison
with the overall population of council households. This
posed no analytical problem in relation to the main purpose
of this study, which centred on the comparison of 'difficult to let' and 'other' areas, but it means that care must
be exercised in analysing the resulting data set in ways
in which this contrast is not centrally employed.

9)   *Classification of all Gateshead EDs*

A cluster analysis based on the same variables was carried
out to classify all the 489 'ordinary' EDs in Gateshead.
This was done in order to interpret the cluster analyses
of the 'council' EDs and the CHAs and to locate them in
the context of Gateshead as a whole. This generated five
distinctive clusters which can be arranged hierarchically
in terms of the 'social space' they represent, and the
location of council housing in the hierarchy. To distinguish these from the CHA clusters the prefix 'ED' will be
used.

The five social'spaces' can be illustrated as follows:

Clusters of all Gateshead EDs

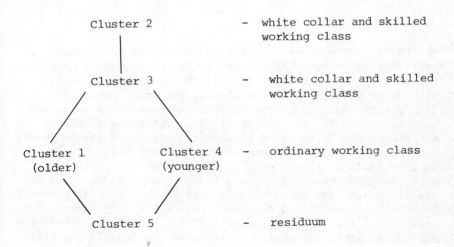

Cluster 2	- white collar and skilled working class
Cluster 3	- white collar and skilled working class
Cluster 1 (older) Cluster 4 (younger)	- ordinary working class
Cluster 5	- residuum

Almost no council EDs were members of ED/Cluster 2, which
scored highest on indicators of affluence, social class and
economic activity. Council housing was well represented in
ED/Cluster 3 which also scored highly on those indicators.
ED/Cluster 3 contained most of what had already been identified as the 'best' council housing but also included some of
the 'intermediate' council housing. ED/Clusters 1 and 4
contained the rest of the 'intermediate' council housing and
the housing purpose built for, or predominantly occupied by,
the elderly, together with much of the pre 1914 private housing in the Borough. ED/Cluster 5 contained overwhelmingly
the 'bad' council housing and is the 'worst' on almost all
indices. The areas in this cluster have the traditional
social characteristics of the 'slum'; almost all consist of
purpose built council housing.

Thus the role of council housing within this hierarchy seems
to be complex. On the one hand it serves for ED/Cluster 5
as a ghetto of the residuum, socially and spatially segregated
into 'difficult to let' estates. On the other hand it is
represented very strongly not only in 'ordinary housing' in
ED/Clusters 1 and 4 but also in the second level of the
hierarchy in ED/Cluster 3.

The five clusters generated from the classification of the 87
CHAs.

Cluster 1 (10 CHAs)

The CHAs in this cluster corresponded closely to estates
generally regarded as 'difficult to let'. Particular features
included a high proportion of children and large households
with a low proportion of the elderly and small households,
high unemployment rates and an over representation of social
classes IV and V. The incidence of single parent families
was almost double that for any other cluster and car ownership
levels were very low. There was a relatively high incidence
of overcrowding, 17 per cent of the households living with
more than one person per room although nearly 40 per cent of
dwellings had five or more rooms. In this cluster 48 per cent
of households contained dependent children. One quarter of
households lived in purpose built flats. Housing turnover was
quite high at 13 per cent. Of the new lettings, 29 per cent
were made for 'living in' families (2), seven per cent were
pensioners and 22 per cent were 'general' transfers. The
number of empty dwellings was at the same level as Clusters
3, 4 and 5. The level of medical transfers out was relatively
high and council house purchase figures very low.

The EDs within the CHAs in this cluster were generally located in ED/Cluster 5.

Cluster 2 (2 CHAs)

This stock clearly had a function as the major current point of entry for new households into local authority tenure. Of all lettings, 71 per cent were to people 'living in'. Children under five were slightly over represented, there were very few pensioners and high proportions of young adults and small households. Unemployment rates were high and coupled with high economic activity for married women, much of which was full time. Given the apparently young character of the population, morbidity rates were surprisingly high. There was an average level of car ownership and an interesting social class composition, with relatively high proportions of social classes II and IV. Over 90 per cent of the stock was purpose built flats, turnover and void rates were very high (35 per cent and 8 per cent respectively). This cluster contained those areas where the practice of the local housing department is to let high rise accommodation in particular to non pensioner single people and young couples without children. Clearly, many first children were from households resident in this stock and spend part of their childhood in it.

The EDs within the CHAs in this cluster were generally located in ED/Cluster 5.

Cluster 3 (14 CHAs)

This can best be described as the 'elderly housing' cluster. There was a very low proportion of children and a high proportion of pensioners. Morbidity indices were relatively high and car ownership rates low. The incidence of single parent families was very low. Nearly two-thirds of the stock consisted of purpose built flats which reflects the housing department's policy of letting a high proportion, particularly of high rise flats, to the middle aged and elderly without children. There were few voids and very little overcrowding. Turnover rates were quite high with a significant proportion of new lettings (13 per cent) made to 'waiting list aged persons' - a category of virtually no importance in any other cluster. The level of council house purchase was low.

The EDs within the CHAs in this cluster were generally located in ED/Cluster 4.

Cluster 4 (38 CHAs)

This was the largest cluster and, overall, is the 'type cluster' for council housing in Gateshead. The population was
generally somewhat older, more manual working class, poorer
and less well housed than is the case for the population of
Gateshead as a whole, but the differences were not very great.
Relatively few lived in purpose built flats, turnover was the
lowest and the level of council house purchase was the highest of all the clusters at 11 per cent. The rate of medical
transfer in either direction was low.

The EDs within the CHAs in this cluster were generally
located in ED/Cluster 1.

Cluster 5 (23 CHAs)

In general terms this seems to be the 'best' council housing
(though 14 per cent of the stock was owner occupied which may
distort the figures to some degree). It resembles Cluster 4
above, the principal differences relating to a higher level
of car ownership and a very high percentage of dwellings with
five or more rooms (64 per cent compared with 34 per cent for
Cluster 4). There was a higher proportion of households with
children (at 39 per cent, second only to Cluster 1) and a high
proportion of heads of households in social class III or above
(especially skilled manual) and a low proportion of flats.

The EDs within the CHAs in this cluster were generally
located in ED/Cluster 3.

Clusters 1 and 2 between them comprised 12 CHAs containing
11,947 people in 4,000 households. These are to be contrasted with the 70,250 people living in 25,475 households in
Clusters 4 and 5. The housing conditions and general social
environment of the two groups are very different although the
intra-group differences are also of interest.

Design and conduct of the survey

The major component of the study comprised the collection and
analysis of data on individuals and households living in public sector housing. This was done by interviewing all individuals (the 'mother figure' in the case of children) in a
sample of households drawn as described above.

Content of the interview

The interview covered four broad areas: housing form (comprising both the type of dwelling itself and the environmental concomitants); housing conditions (the size and density of occupation, the physical condition and amenities of the dwelling and its surroundings and the attitudes to it of the inhabitants); health and ill health (including details of temporary and long standing illnesses; their effects on daily living and the use of medical services); and other relevant factors (age, sex, occupation, income, housing history and smoking and drinking habits). In order to operationalise the four main elements, the researchers looked for guidance to other studies. The Department of the Environment's, National Dwelling and Housing Survey (1979b, 1980a) and English House Condition Survey (1978, 1979a, 1982, 1983), the General Household Survey (OPCS, annual), Townsend's, Poverty in the United Kingdom (1979), the Medical Research Council's approved questionnaire on respiratory symptoms (1976), the National Study of the Health and Growth of Schoolchildren (undated) and Brown and Harris's, The Social Origins of Depression (1978) were especially helpful. Using other studies as a starting point has positive advantages in terms of the comparability of data especially for a geographically limited pilot study such as this.

Given the central focus of the study, the relationship between housing and health, there was a particular interest in those 'illnesses' known, or suspected of being, associated with poor housing. Thus respondents were asked in some detail about respiratory disease, rheumatic/arthritic conditions, depressive illnesses and, in the case of children, accidents. Health was also more directly linked with housing by asking respondents whether they perceived any relationships.

Structure of the interviews

The interview schedules were mainly structured, although open ended questions were used to explore attitudes and feelings. Where questions were open ended or classification could be complex (e.g. occupation, illnesses), responses were recorded verbatim and post coded. Questions were kept as non technical as possible. Five interview schedules were developed; these were:

a) *Housing information schedule:* Administered to the initial adult contact. It asked straightforward questions about housing.

b) *Housing conditions and family health schedule:* Administer-
    ed to the 'mother figure' in households with children,
    otherwise to the initial adult contact. It asked more
    detailed questions on housing and environs, attitudes
    to these and any effects on the health of household
    members.

c) *Health schedule for children:* Administered to the 'mother
    figure'. It asked questions about health and the use of
    medical services.

d) *Individual health and employment schedule for adults:*
    Administered to each adult. It asked questions about
    health, use of medical services, smoking, drinking, emplo-
    yment and employment history and income.

e) *Self-administered questionnaire on health and employment:*
    Left for adults with whom interviewers were unable to make
    contact. The questionnaire was a contracted version of
    d) above.

Pilot study

The pilot study consisted of interviews with the members of
households, conducted by the researchers. Following the pilot
study minor modifications were made to the interview schedules
and strategies devised for coping with callback visits,
refusals and interview management.

Main survey

Most of the interviewing was conducted in a four week period in
May and June 1983. Fifteen interviewers were recruited and,
after two days training, two were allocated to each of seven
CHAs and one to the remaining CHA. Special attention was given
in preparing interviewers for the plethora of responses they
would be likely to receive regarding the section on the
schedules relating to income, especially state benefits, which
were complicated by recent changes such as the introduction of
employers' sick-pay. A room was hired in Gateshead as a
centre for interviewers, with at least one member of the
research team in attendance each weekday morning; interviewers were expected to visit the centre at least twice each week.

All 480 households sampled received an introductory letter
prior to being approached by an interviewer. Strategies such
as leaving cards and self-administered questionnaires were
used where it proved difficult to contact households or
individual members of households.

Response rate

Of the 480 households in the sample interviews were conducted
with all the members of 353 (74 per cent) and with some of
the members of 30 (6 per cent). Interviewers were unable to
contact 35 households (7 per cent) and the remaining 62 households (13 per cent) declined to participate. There was some
variation in the 'success rates' between estates (65-93 per
cent). These response rates compare favourably with other
surveys which attempt to interview all household members.
Townsend claims that his study achieved complete interviews in
75 per cent of households (1979). The 1981 GHS (1983) achieved a response to all sections of the survey of 72 per cent.

The refusal rate, at 13 per cent, is not excessively high.
Townsend (1979) and the 1981 GHS (1983) reported 15.6 per cent
and 12 per cent respectively. Non-contacts, at seven per
cent are higher than either of these surveys (Townsend
reported 1.9 per cent and GHS, 2 per cent) and might have
been reduced by a longer interviewing period. However, the
main reason for a relatively high level of non-contact was
the high incidence in the sample of property with a high rate
of turnover and a tendency for property to remain empty for
some time following termination of tenancy.

Coding

A number of part time coders were employed to check the pre-
coded responses and to post code the open ended responses.
Health conditions were coded according to 18 categories
designed for the International Classification of Health
Problems in Primary Health Care (1979). Occupations and ind-
ustries were coded using the 1981 Census coding index (OPCS,
1980).

All responses to each of the remaining open ended questions
were listed and from these, appropriate categories were derived. Multiple response was accounted for by assigning a column
to each response category and coding '1' if a category applied
and 'O' if it did not. The coded schedules were transferred
to a computer data file which was used to create an SPSS
archive file containing 902 cases and 691 variables.

NOTES

(1) Housing form: the complex of dwelling type and general
     environment. The dwelling types identified were: semi-
     detached house; terraced house, low rise flats and maison-

ettes (traditional); medium rise flats and maisonettes
(traditional); medium rise flats and maisonettes (system-
built); high rise flats.

(2) 'Living in' : separate families who have applied for local
authority housing on the grounds that they are forced to
live with another family. In Census terms they may be
part of the same household but they wish to establish a
separate household.

4 The sample of households and the analysis of the findings

The previous chapter discussed the issues which influenced the methods chosen for the 'housing and health' study, the way in which the housing areas were selected and also the research procedures that were used.

This chapter will discuss the research on which the book is based in greater detail. It is divided into three sections. The first of these will set out the characteristics of the sample of households and those of the individuals living within the households. The second section will compare the main findings with recent national data, drawn largely from the GHS and the NDHS. In the third, and largest, section the findings of the study will be reported: differences between the eight housing areas will be identified by focusing on specific factors, namely; housing defects, environmental defects, dissatisfaction with housing and residents' perceptions of relationships between housing and health.

Positive and negative effects of particular policies will be referred to: the former in relation to the medical priority transfer system which counters some of the outcomes of bad housing, especially for elderly people; the latter with reference to the sale of council housing which, by reducing the stock available for letting discriminates against those living in 'difficult to let' housing.

Stage 1

The primary purpose of the study was to compare housing conditions and health in different types of housing areas. In
order to be able to make comparisons it was necessary to
ensure that a reasonable number of households were included in
the sample from each housing area. To do this equal numbers
of households in eight distinct housing areas were sampled.
This sampling approach facilitates the making of comparisons,
but does not provide a sample representative of the population, unless the sampling units are equivalent in size.

In Gateshead, the clusters from which housing areas were
selected are distinctly variable in size; they ranged from
662 households in Cluster 2 to 16,758 households in Cluster
5. The effect of this kind of disproportionate sampling is
that characteristics of the smaller sampling units become
over-represented in the final sample. Some of the effects of
this can be observed in Table 4.1 which compares certain census indicators relating to all Gateshead EDs with 'council'
EDs and the aggregate of the eight housing areas selected in
the first stage of sampling.

Table 4.1
Comparison of Gateshead EDs, council EDs and
the selected CHAs using nine census indicators

	All Gateshead E.Ds.	Council E.Ds.	Eight CHAs in sample
% Purpose built flats	14.4	18.7	35.1
% Households density > 1 person per room	5.0	7.2	10.4
% Households with children	32.8	31.5	40.0
% Single-parent households	4.9	6.7	10.0
% Large households (6+ persons)	3.3	4.7	6.5
% Single person households	23.0	25.2	22.5
% Households with no car	57.8	71.3	76.0
% Households with two cars	6.8	3.3	2.3
% Households with 5+ rooms	46.8	39.4	41.4

The data in Table 4.1 suggests that the housing areas which emerged from the first stage of sampling are not representative of a population of all Gateshead housing or even of all Gateshead council housing. The sample housing areas differ from all housing and all council housing in the following respects:

a)   a greater proportion of purpose built flats.

b)   more overcrowding.

c)   more large households.

d)   more households with children.

e)   more single parent households.

f)   less car ownership.

Put simply, the effect is over representation of disadvantaged households living in the least favourable housing conditions. Consequently one would expect higher levels of poor health than in a representative sample of Gateshead council housing. However, the primary purpose of the survey was not to obtain a sample which would provide unbiased estimates of population parameters, nor was it to determine the prevalence of bad housing and poor health in Gateshead per se. No suggestion is made that Gateshead itself is an unhealthy place in which to live; that is another story. The primary purpose was to show variation in housing conditions and self assessed health and a relationship between them. Thus the sample with potentially wide variation in housing and environmental type served the purpose.

Stage 2

The survey itself involved interviews with members of 383 households which were located in eight randomly selected housing areas. Equal numbers of households were sampled in each of the housing areas but there proved to be differential rates of response, ranging from 75 per cent in St Cuthberts and Wrekenton to 95 per cent in Meadow Lane. Every adult member was interviewed in all but 20 of the households. The total number of persons about whom information was collected was 902 (674 adults and 228 children). Table 4.2 shows the number of households and the number of individuals by CHA.

As was the case with households, the number of responses received from individuals varied from area to area. This was partly due to differences in response rates among households but more importantly, due to differences in demographic structures of the areas. St Cuthberts and Old Fold were selected from 'clusters' of housing areas characterised by high

Table 4.2

Numbers of households and numbers of individuals by CHA

CHA	No. of households	No. of individuals
St Cuthberts	45	147
Old Fold	50	153
Nursery Lane	46	90
Carlisle Court	47	96
Wrekenton	45	120
Beacon Lough	47	130
Allerdene	46	57
Meadow Lane	57	109
All CHAs	383	902

proportions of children in the population. Consequently over
half of the children in the sample came from these two housing
areas. Proportions of children in housing areas varied between zero in Allerdene to 43 per cent in St Cuthberts. The
distribution of adults was also determined by structural
factors to some extent. There were least adults in Nursery
Lane and Allerdene, which contained 10 per cent and eight per
cent respectively of all adults in the sample. These areas
were both characterised by relatively high proportions of
single person households. Housing areas with large numbers of
adults were Beacon Lough, Wrekenton and Old Fold (15 per cent,
14 per cent and 14 per cent respectively). These are all low
rise estates which consist specifically of family accommodation; high numbers of adults result from intact families and/
or grown up children.

Table 4.3. shows the type of housing occupied by households
which participated in the survey. Three housing areas are
entirely medium to high rise - St Cuthberts, Nursery Lane and
Allerdene. Carlisle Court is predominantly medium rise but
does contain some houses, bungalows and low rise flats. Old
Fold, Wrekenton, Beacon Lough and Meadow Lane are all low rise
housing areas although they contain varying amounts of flats.
These flats are all in two storey blocks which usually contain
only four flats (two up and two down). They tend to be identical in external appearance to adjoining semi detached housing.

Comparison of the 1982 GHS (1984) households and those in
the 'housing and health' study show some differences.

74

Table 4.3
Type of housing occupied by households

	Bungalow	House	Flats low rise	Flats & Maisonettes medium to high rise	Total
St Cuthberts	–	–	–	45	45
Old Fold	5	44	1	–	50
Nursery Lane	–	–	–	46	46
Carlisle Court	3	6	1	37	47
Wrekenton	6	30	9	–	45
Beacon Lough	9	28	10	–	47
Allerdene	–	–	–	46	46
Meadow Lane	13	20	24	–	57
All CHAs	36	128	45	174	383

Of the 1982 GHS (1984) respondents, 32 per cent of households contained children under 16, 23 per cent were single
person households, 12 per cent were single parent households,
three per cent of households contained six or more persons and
two per cent lived at a density of more than one person per
room. Overall, in the 'housing and health' sample around one-
third of all households contained children under 16, but this
varied from none in Allerdene to nearly two-thirds in St
Cuthberts. Conversely, while 36 per cent of the total sample
consisted of single person households, this ranged from seven
per cent in St Cuthberts to 78 per cent in Allerdene. Only
five per cent of the households were headed by single parents;
the highest proportion was located in St. Cuthberts where 13
per cent of households were headed by a single parent. These
figures are low compared to census data relating to the housing areas and single parent households appear to be under-
represented. Large households and overcrowding also appeared
to be relatively uncommon. Only four per cent of households
contained six or more persons and the same proportion were
living at a density of more than one person per room. In two
housing areas - St Cuthberts and Old Fold - more than one in
10 households were overcrowded and around the same proportion
(presumably mostly the same households) contained six or more
persons.

There appeared to be significantly less overcrowding among
the Old Fold sample than in the housing area as a whole;
census data showed that 25 per cent of households in the Old
Fold housing area lived at a density of one or more persons
per room, though only 12 per cent lived in large households
(6 or more persons).

Of the 674 adults in the sample, 131 (19 per cent) were aged
over 65 years, a slightly higher proportion than the 15 per
cent recorded by the 1982 GHS (1984). Over half the elderly
lived in either Allerdene (30 per cent) or Meadow Lane (26 per
cent). Allerdene, in this respect, proved to be an extreme
form of its parent cluster; census figures show that 71 per
cent of this housing area were aged over 65 years, while the
corresponding figure for the cluster from which the housing
area was selected is 43 per cent. The modal ages of adults
were 16-24 years old in Nursery Lane, 25-44 years old in
St Cuthberts, Old Fold and Beacon Lough, 45-64 years old in
Carlisle Court and Wrekenton and over 65 years old in Allerdene and Meadow Lane.

The sex distribution of the sample compared very closely
with that of the 1982 GHS (1984) sample. There were more
females (474) than males (428) in the 'housing and health'
study, i.e. 53 per cent and 47 per cent respectively, compared with 52 per cent and 48 per cent respectively recorded by
GHS. This was mainly due to the high presence of females
among the over 65 group (72 out of 131). Over half of the
adults in the sample were married, one-quarter were single,
15 per cent widowed and eight per cent divorced or separated.
Differences between housing areas were marked, due partly to
differences in age structure. Thus, over half of those from
Allerdene were widowed. Beacon Lough contained the highest
proportion of married adults (66 per cent) while over one-
quarter of those from Nursery Lane were divorced or separated.

One-quarter of the adults in the sample were employed,
around one-quarter were keeping house, over one-fifth were
unemployed and just under one-fifth were retired. There were
small proportions in full time education (2 per cent) and
permanently sick (4 per cent). The larger categories again
reflected the variation between housing areas. In Carlisle
Court, Wrekenton and Beacon Lough over 40 per cent of adults
were in full time employment, in Allerdene over half were
retired and in St Cuthberts approaching 40 per cent were keeping house. Carlisle Court had a significantly low proportion
of 'housekeepers' (12 per cent). Of course this category is
somewhat ill defined and depends on how many elderly women
define themselves as retired as well as on the employment
opportunities for younger married women. High 'housekeeping'

76

figures for St Cuthberts (37 per cent) and Old Fold (28 per cent) compared to, say, Beacon Lough (17 per cent) take on more meaning when reported unemployment is considered. Unemployment was much higher in St Cuthberts (31 per cent), Old Fold (33 per cent) and Nursery Lane (55 per cent); for the five remaining housing areas unemployment averaged seven per cent. In Nursery Lane over four in every five adults were either unemployed or keeping house.

Male unemployment varied considerably from area to area. Table 4.4 shows the proportion of unemployed, economically active males, by CHA.

Table 4.4

Proportion of economically active males unemployed by CHA

CHA	% unemployed
St Cuthberts	80
Old Fold	71
Nursery Lane	89
Carlisle Court	27
Wrekenton	21
Beacon Lough	42
Allerdene	17
Meadow Lane	21

Discounting Allerdene which had few economically active males, the range was from 21 per cent in Meadow Lane and Wrekenton to 71 per cent in Old Fold, 80 per cent in St Cuthberts and 89 per cent in Nursery Lane. Male unemployment in the sample was a considerable overestimate of what would be expected from census results, where it was 45 per cent in St Cuthberts, 49 per cent in Old Fold and 32 per cent in Nursery Lane. This discrepancy may be due to response bias - people in employment are more difficult to catch at home - or may reflect rising levels of unemployment during the two year period between the census and the survey. In April 1981, 58,891 males were registered as unemployed in the Tyne and Wear Metropolitan County. By April 1983 this had increased to 71,019, an increase of 20 per cent. (Department of Employment, 1981, 1983).

A consequence of high unemployment was that 386 individuals lived in households which were totally dependent on state benefits for family finance; 327 of these lived in non-pensioner households. Of those from non-pensioner households

75 per cent lived in St Cuthberts, Nursery Lane or Old Fold. Each of these housing areas was characterised by relatively large proportions of persons living in 'state dependent' households; St Cuthberts (72 per cent), Nursery Lane (70 per cent) and Old Fold (57 per cent).

HOUSING AND HEALTH:COMPARISONS WITH NATIONAL DATA

In setting up this exploratory study and, more particularly, in constructing the interview schedules for the survey of households, it was decided that wherever possible information should be collected in such a way as to facilitate comparisons with other studies and surveys.

This has a number of advantages. It enables an assessment of how far the sample was similar to, or differed from, those of other surveys along a variety of dimensions. If a number of studies collect comparable data, it enables the building-up of information relating to the area of research and the confirmation or requestioning of previous findings. Last, but not least, it is useful in a pragmatic sense to utilise questions and ways of collecting information which have already been 'tried and tested'. Data from two government studies will be considered here: the General Household Survey (OPCS, annual) and the National Dwelling and Housing Survey 1978 (DoE 1979b). The comparison will focus on two areas of particular interest to the present study: housing and health/illness, together with some reference to employment status.

The General Household Survey (GHS) is conducted annually although the questions asked and the analyses conducted vary somewhat from year to year. It provided a model for the present study in questions relating to some aspects of housing, to health , illness and the use of medical services, to smoking and drinking habits and to employment and income. Thus it is possible to compare the findings in a number of areas. There are, of course, many limitations to the comparison. The surveys are very different - GHS (1982) involves interviewing the adult members of over 10,000 households, compared with 383 households in the 1983 'housing and health' study which is the subject of this book, and the age, sex and social class distribution of the individuals involved in the GHS report is more akin to that of the population as a whole. In addition, between 1982 and 1983, some significant changes occurred, particularly related to unemployment. Where possible, comparisons are made with the GHS carried out in 1982, but, in some cases analyses are only available for earlier years.

The 1978 National Dwelling and Household Survey (NDHS) offers a detailed picture of housing conditions in a sample of
local authority areas in England although the figures are now
some years out of date. It did not provide a model for
questions as did the GHS, but it is of particular interest
as one of the sample areas was Gateshead. Thus it is possible
to compare the housing conditions experienced by the 'housing
and health' sample of households with those of Gateshead as a
whole in 1977 and also to see how Gateshead stood in relation
to the overall sample of local authority areas. All the NDHS
figures in this section relate to the Gateshead sample.

Housing

While all of the households interviewed in the 'housing and
health' study lived in council built accommodation (and all
but 3.1 per cent in council owned accommodation), the proportion of households in the NDHS Gateshead sample who were council tenants was 48.2 per cent (DoE, 1979b). This was higher
than the national average of 30 per cent with a correspondingly lower proportion of owner occupiers (37 per cent compared
to 54 per cent). Thus, renting from the council is the
dominant tenure in Gateshead and was the experience of nearly
half of all Gateshead households surveyed by NDHS. However,
this means that the following discussion involves a comparison
of the housing conditions of a sample of 383 households all
living in council property in 1983 with those of a sample of
nearly 83,000 households, over half of whom do not live in
council property in 1977.

In terms of accommodation, there are substantial differences
between the households surveyed and Gateshead as a whole,
reflecting the far greater importance in the public sector of
flats and maisonettes. Whereas in 1977 NDHS found that three-
quarters of households lived in detached, semi detached or
terraced houses, this only applied to about 43 per cent of the
households in the 'housing and health' study. Fifty six per
cent lived in flats and maisonettes. This difference is
reflected in differences between the proportion of households
living above ground level. The NDHS households overwhemingly
lived in accommodation where the lowest floor was at ground
or lower than ground level (84.8 per cent) while this only
applied to 59 per cent of the 'housing and health' households.
Over one-quarter of the 'housing and health' study households
(many of them containing elderly people) lived on the third
floor or above.

The dwellings of the households in the 'housing and health' study also tended to have fewer rooms than those of Gateshead as a whole. NDHS found that over half the households surveyed in Gateshead had five or more rooms, while this only applied to five per cent of 'housing and health' households. The proportion of households with three or fewer rooms were, respectively, 11.3 per cent and 61.9 per cent. There were corresponding differences in the number of bedrooms, but not nearly to the same extent. Thus, it seems that the differences lay in living space more than bedrooms. However, the boundary between these is not fixed - a household may well utilise a living room if an extra bedroom is needed.

The smaller size of dwellings is not simply associated with the 'housing and health' households containing a smaller number of persons. In that study, there was a greater proportion of one person households, but a smaller proportion of two person households who, if they consisted of a married couple, could be considered to need very similar sized accommodation to one person. It seems that in this sense, public sector housing in Gateshead is more heavily utilised and less under-occupied than the private stock. Of course, the six year gap between the two studies may be significant here, as the public sector has increasingly provided small dwellings for small, elderly households.

The findings confirmed the impression of less under occupation. While nearly 80 per cent of Gateshead households in the NDHS survey were living at a density of less than 0.75 persons per room, this applied to only around 70 per cent in the 'housing and health' study. While there was little evidence of serious overcrowding in the latter study, 12 per cent were living at a density of one or more persons per room, compared with just over three per cent of NDHS households.

Turning to the amenities possessed by the dwellings, the NDHS found that by 1977 over 95 per cent of the Gateshead households had sole use of all basic amenities. The likelihood is that since 1977 the proportion has increased further, approaching the 100 per cent figure in the 'housing and health' survey.

Central heating provides an indicator of housing conditions which is perhaps more relevant for contemporary studies. As with the traditional basic amenities, it appears that the public sector is relatively well provided for. Only four per cent of households in the 'housing and health' study had no central heating, compared with over one-third (36.4 per cent) in the NDHS. This figure was lower than the national average (47 per cent with no central heating), perhaps reflecting the higher proportion of public sector dwellings. This is an area where the gap of six years between the two studies is likely to be important. By 1982, GHS found the proportion of households with central heating nationally had reached 60 per cent (OPCS, 1984, Table 5.3).

However, it can be argued persuasively that central heating can only be described as an amenity if the occupants of the dwelling are willing and able to meet the costs incurred. Indeed, if it is assumed in the design and construction of houses that the heating system installed will be used, expensive and unpopular forms of central heating could be described as a 'disamenity'. The household faces the alternatives of incurring high heating bills or risking condensation and other dampness problems. The main form of room heating used by different households was explored in both surveys. Although over 96 per cent of households in the 'housing and health' study had central heating, only 57 per cent used it as their main form of room heating. On the other hand, while only about 64 per cent of the NDHS households had central heating, over 55 per cent used this as their main form of room heating. These differences are likely to stem from a mixture of differences in the economic circumstances of the households surveyed and also from differences in the type of central heating system. Gas central heating was by far the most popular form of heating among NDHS respondents compared to electric central heating which was the most common type found in the public sector housing of the 'housing and health' study (electric heating being relatively cheap to install but often expensive to run and sometimes inefficient). In the 1981 GHS (1983) survey gas central heating was also the most popular type of heating (37 per cent), electricity being used by only 17 per cent of those with central heating (10 per cent of the sample) and it was those using electric heating who were least likely to use it as their main form of room heating in the winter.

It is also possible to compare some of the characteristics of the respondents in the 'housing and health' study and NDHS, as well as characteristics of the dwellings in which they lived. In both studies, economically active respondents were classified by socio economic group - one indicator of class membership. As expected, the 'housing and health' study contained fewer professional and other non manual workers (22 per cent compared with 39 per cent) and more semi and unskilled manual workers (49 per cent compared with 29 per cent). The proportion of skilled manual workers in the two studies was almost identical at a little over 30 per cent. It is worth noting that nine per cent of the economically active respondents in the 'housing and health' study had never worked. Presumably these are included in the three per cent classified as 'other' in the NDHS since the category 'never worked' was not specified. While allowing for differences in the composition of the two samples, this is likely to be mainly attributable to the deteriorating employment situation between 1977 and 1983.

Comparing the length of time that households had been resident at their current address, the NDHS households were somewhat more likely to have been resident there for 10 or more years and somewhat less likely to have moved within the last two years than those in the 'housing and health' study. However, overall the impression is not of a highly mobile population. Almost four out of 10 households in the 'housing and health' study had not moved within the last 10 years.

Both the NDHS and the 'housing and health' study also looked at three indicators of satisfaction which related to housing, viz: attitudes of households to the number of rooms in the dwelling, their satisfaction with the dwelling and their satisfaction with the surrounding environment. The questions were phrased somewhat differently in the two studies, but were similar enough to enable comparison.

Overall, the responses show a lesser degree of satisfaction in relation to both dwelling itself and the surrounding environment among the council house respondents of the 'housing and health' study. This is least marked in relation to the number of rooms. In relation to the dwelling and its surrounds, around 80 per cent of NDHS households were recorded as 'very satisfied' or 'satisfied', compared with only about 63 per cent of 'housing and health' study households. Dissatisfaction was expressed by over one-quarter of the latter households compared with only about 12 per cent of those in NDHS. These differences may reflect a number of factors, for example, differences in objective conditions or differences in attitudes towards property which is owner occupied and that which belongs to someone else (the local authority) and to which the household has been allocated, possibly with a limited degree of choice. However, the 'housing and health' study was deliberately constructed to include some 'bad' council housing. Breakdown of responses by estates showed that dissatisfaction was chiefly expressed by those living in this 'bad' housing, suggesting that objective conditions rather than attitudes to public sector rented accommodation is the crucial factor (see pp. 92-93).

Health and illness

One major area of interest for both the 1982 GHS (1984) and
the present study is that of health and illness and it is of
particular interest to see how the 'housing and health' sample
of households compared to the national pattern in terms of
various indices of self reported morbidity. According to
certain indices, the present sample emerged as in considerably
worse health. Many more reported their health over the last
12 months as 'not good' (26 per cent compared with 13 per
cent), and many fewer as 'good' (44 per cent compared with 59
per cent). A higher percentage reported some long standing
illness (37 per cent compared with 30 per cent) but differences were especially marked in relation to reported acute sickness. In 1982, the GHS found 10 per cent of males and 13 per
cent of females reported illness during the last two weeks.
The corresponding figures for the present study were 24 per
cent for males and 34 per cent for females.

Other indices of morbidity are not so easy to compare, as
the questions in the two studies were not worded in exactly
the same way. For example, there were some questions relating to the use of medical services. The GHS asked respondents
about all consultations with their general practitioner (GP),
including those by telephone, over the last two weeks, whereas
the present study asked respondents whether they had visited
or been visited by their GP in the last month. The proportions reporting consultations were 11 per cent (males) and 15
per cent (females) in the GHS and 33 per cent (males and
females) in the 'housing and health' study. The GHS found
that 12 per cent of males and females had attended the casu-
alty or outpatient department of a hospital during the last
three months. The present study found 11 per cent of respondents had attended over the last month.

The 1981 GHS asked in some detail about the health and
abilities of respondents aged 65 and over and some comparison
with the 'housing and health' study is possible for that age
group. The findings are striking. While respondents in the
latter study reported less difficulty than GHS respondents
with sight and hearing, when they were asked about limitations
on their abilities to do certain things, they reported
considerably more difficulty along virtually all comparable
dimensions. The only exception was cooking a main meal,
which the present study found was least related to age. Thus,
for example, 49 per cent of the 'housing and health' sample
reported difficulties in 'climbing stairs', whereas only eight
per cent of GHS respondents reported difficulty in 'getting up
and down stairs and steps'. This may partly be accounted for by

the fact that nearly half of the elderly respondents in the present study lived off the ground floor (see p. 76). However, other discrepancies are less easy to explain. For example, 29 per cent of the present sample found difficulty in 'bathing, showering or washing all over' (GHS 9 per cent); 32 per cent found it difficult to 'do household shopping' (GHS 14 per cent) 55 per cent found it difficult to 'do heavy housework' (GHS 10 per cent to sweep or clean floors and 17 per cent to wash inside windows). The elderly in the 'housing and health' study came from the lower end of the social class structure and may contain some over representation of the older elderly, but the size of these differences seems to reveal some real differences in functional incapacity.

Overall, in relation to these indices, respondents in the 'housing and health' study reported consistently higher levels of morbidity than did the GHS respondents. The over representation of older people in the former population could account for much of this difference. However, there are some features which may merit further consideration. For example, one of the most striking differences was in reported recent acute illness, which one would not expect to be as strongly related to growing older as, for example, the presence of long standing illness. Considerably greater limitations on functional capacities were reported by respondents aged 65 and over in the 'housing and health' study than in the GHS.

Smoking and drinking

Many of the questions in the 'housing and health' study about smoking and drinking were derived from the GHS.

Respondents appeared to be more likely to smoke than the GHS sample; 70 per cent were or had been smokers compared with 58 per cent of GHS respondents. More were current cigarette smokers (49 per cent compared with 35 per cent). Comparing the number of cigarettes smoked in a day, 'housing and health' respondents were also heavier smokers, 11 per cent of these smoking less than 10 cigarettes a day compared with 19 per cent in the GHS.

On the other hand, 'housing and health' respondents reported that they were less likely to drink alcohol. Thirty per cent said that they never had a drink nowadays, compared with only nine per cent of respondents in the GHS. This may result from the larger proportion of elderly in the former study. Those in the present study who did drink, however, seemed to drink somewhat more - for example, only 17 per cent said that they 'hardly drink at all', compared with 34 per cent in the GHS.

Both surveys also asked people whether they thought smoking and drinking could damage health. Responses in relation to drinking alcohol were broadly similar (more than one-third of each sample). However, the 'housing and health' respondents seemed more optimistic about the effects of smoking. For example, while four-fifths of GHS respondents gave an unqualified 'yes' in response to the question 'do you think that smoking can damage people's health?' only two-thirds of the former respondents did so.

Employment and income

The 'housing and health' study used many of the same questions as the GHS in relation to employment and income. However, these are areas in which comparison is particularly difficult, not only because of the different ways of drawing the sample of households, but also because of the one year difference in the timing of the surveys. Employment and income data are particularly affected by this gap, during which unemployment increased rapidly and inflation altered the real value of money. The 1982 GHS notes the marked decline in economic activity rates over the previous decade, especially among men, and the marked increase in unemployment (OPCS, 1984, p.93).

These differences are immediately evident if one looks at the responses to questions about employment status over the last week. Even in 1982 a sample of the population drawn from Gateshead council housing would have presented a rather different picture from that of GHS data for the whole country. By 1983, the differences, remembering too the higher proportion of elderly in the 'housing and health' sample, are enormous. While 54 per cent of adult respondents in the 1981 GHS reported that they had a job, only 28 per cent of the present sample did so. Twenty two per cent were unemployed in the 'housing and health' study compared with six per cent in the GHS and nearly half were economically inactive, compared with 23 per cent in the GHS.

The scale and nature of the differences between the surveys prevent any meaningful comparisons of household income. Given that the respondents in the 'housing and health' study were drawn from a sector of the housing market which has increasingly tended to accommodate the poorer groups in society (Forrest and Murie, 1983) and from a part of the country where incomes tend to be lower on average (Central Statistical Office CSO - 1984, Table 8.4) and unemployment higher than average (CSO, 1984, Table 7.13), it is likely that their household incomes were lower than those of GHS respondents. Elsewhere, it has been noted that there was a very high degree of dependence on state means tested benefits and that this was not only attributable to the over representation of the elderly in the sample.

'HOUSING AND HEALTH' SURVEY: ANALYSIS OF FINDINGS

Introduction

The study was primarily concerned with examining the extent to which self assessed health varies between different sets of housing circumstances. Initial analysis was concerned with identification of differences between eight housing areas, which were randomly selected from eight area types, generated by a two-stage cluster analysis of census enumeration districts. The indicators of health which were employed in the analysis were measured on either dichotomous or ordinal scales. In effect, the dichotomous variables could also be described as ordinal; if questions are asked about the presence of illnesses then clearly those who answer 'yes' can be ranked as more ill than those who answer 'no'.

In some cases responses have been combined to construct cumulative indicants. Where possible, reliability of these derived scales has been estimated by employing Cronbach's alpha, which is a measure of internal consistency (Cronbach, 1951). Reliability of a scale refers to the extent to which repeated measurement would give equivalent scores. But scales also require validity, which refers to the extent to which they can be said to measure what they are supposed to measure, and is usually more difficult to assess. One way to estimate validity is to calculate the extent to which scales correlate with other items designed to measure the same phenomenon. This relates to construct validity which Zeller and Carmines (1980) suggest:

> ...focuses on the assessment of whether a particular
> measure relates to other measures consistent with
> theoretically derived hypotheses concerning the
> concepts (or constructs) that are measured. (p. 81)

When responses were on a yes/no dichotomy, analysis was usually conducted via chi-square procedures. Where measurement was on ordinal scales, the analysis of ridits techniques developed by Bross (1958) was usually employed. The results of ridit analysis are presented as pictorial representations of confidence estimates, which enables comparisons to be made between two or more sampling units. In the confidence interval diagrams (e.g. see Fig. 4.1) the horizontal line at 0.5 represents the sample average; where a confidence interval does not overlap this horizontal line, a sampling unit may be regarded as significantly different from the sample average. Where confidence intervals for sampling units do not overlap each other they may be considered to be significantly different.

The alphabetic codes used in certain ridit analysis diagrams have the following relationship with housing areas:

A	-	St Cuthberts
B	-	Old Fold
C	-	Nursery Lane
D	-	Carlisle Court
E	-	Wrekenton
F	-	Beacon Lough
G	-	Allerdene
H	-	Meadow Lane

As an example of interpretation of ridit analysis results, consider Figure 4.1 - ridit analysis of dampness. Housing areas A and B have significantly higher scores on the dampness index than the sample average. Housing areas F and H score less than the sample average. Housing area A is significantly damper than all housing areas except B and C. Housing area B is significantly damper than F, G and H. Housing area C is significantly damper than housing area H.

Simple comparisons between housing areas do not present any major problems. However, the unique contribution which housing circumstances make to states of health can be difficult to disentangle. Health states may be related to several factors which may themselves be associated with housing circumstances - e.g. social class, income, sex, diet, smoking, drinking and employment. As far as this study was concerned, the major objectives were to analyse and account for the differences in self assessed health, between types of housing and housing areas and to explore the network of relationships between housing, health and various related factors. Therefore, most of the analysis is exploratory; there was less concern with the rigorous testing of specific hypotheses than with observing patterns and connections within the data which suggested explanations of any health differences between individuals, especially where health differences were associated with housing differences.

Most of the data collected for this survey was at an ordinal or lower level of measurement and therefore lends itself to non-parametric techniques. However, exploration of inter-variate relationships requires some form of multi-variate analysis. In this situation chi-square and ridit analysis are limited or unwieldy (or both). If ridit analysis or chi-square are used, controlling for sex and five socio economic categories, 10 separate analyses will be required; besides being unwieldy this tends to result in extremely small (or zero) frequencies in some sampling units.

Log-linear and logit analysis would be one way of dealing with this level of data and log-linear methods were used to a limited extent. However, the flexibility and comparative simplicity of parametric methods was preferred. There have been long running debates about the nature of the relationship between measurement and statistical techniques (1). The decision to ignore measurement restrictions does not indicate support of the 'measurement independent' position which states that statistical techniques and measurement considerations are independent of each other. Parametric techniques were used purely for pragmatic reasons; because to do so provided great-er flexibility in manipulation of the data. Some useful insights regarding patterns of inter-variate relationships were gained by using techniques such as multiple regression and analysis of variance, which could only be employed by ignoring assumptions related to levels of measurements.

Housing defects

There are two possible approaches to the survey of housing conditions; one is on the spot assessment by experts - as in the English House Condition Survey. The other is investigat-ion of the perceptions of the occupants of dwellings. On the spot assessment demands considerable expertise and is consequently expensive to conduct, thus the second option was used and the opinions of occupants sought. What a person feels about the housing conditions in which he or she lives can be as relevant, to subsequent health states, as objective assessment by independent experts. Furthermore, expert assessment tends to relate to observation at a particular point in time, certain housing conditions (e.g. dampness) do not remain constant. Only a person who occupies a dwelling for a period of time can really know what it is like to live in it.

Perceptions of housing conditions were elicited, first of all, by asking, 'Is there anything wrong with the structure of this dwelling?' If the answer was positive, the question, 'What are the defects?' was asked, followed by, 'Is it a serious defect or only minor?' and 'Does it affect the health of you and your family?'. Through this approach it was intended to obtain responses regarding defects which were in the immediate consciousness of respondents. This was then followed by prompting, mentioning particular defects, and asking if the dwelling had each of them.

e.g.   'Does your dwelling have rising damp, damp walls or ceilings?'

'Is it serious or minor?'

'Does it affect the health of you or your family?'.

It was found that 57 per cent of households complained about ill fitting doors and windows, 43 per cent lived in dwellings which were described as damp and 23 per cent complained about flaking paint. Other structural defects mentioned included loose brickwork and plaster, broken floor boards, damaged staircases and leaking roofs.

Analysis of positive responses to each of the items revealed a relationship between housing conditions and housing location. St Cuthberts' residents reported the greatest frequency of housing defects, with dampness especially prevalent. Old Fold had most reports of damaged brickwork and plaster, broken floor boards and flaking paint - clearly this prewar property was considered to be in need of refurbishment. Nursery Lane had the greatest frequency of ill fitting doors and windows and hence, the associated problem of draughts.

Thus, the greatest frequency of housing defects occurred in those housing areas with the most deprived social conditions - St Cuthberts, Nursery Lane and Old Fold - the three housing areas made up of estates defined by the local authority as 'difficult to let'.

The questionnaire items relating to housing defects were employed to construct cumulative indicants. Scores were assigned as follows:

If defect present: score 1

If defect serious: add 1

If defect affects
 health   : add 1

If defect was
 mentioned unprompted: add 1

89

Thus for each defect there was a scale of seriousness ranging from O to 4. The two most frequently mentioned were then subjected to ridit analysis. The results of this are shown in Figure 4.1, and indicate that St Cuthberts and Old Fold were both significantly worse than the mean in terms of severity of dampness. Beacon Lough and Meadow Lane were both significantly better than average, although some respondents in Beacon Lough did complain about leaking roofs. Nursery Lane had the third worst rate of dampness although it was not significantly worse than the sample mean. On the other hand, Nursery Lane was the one housing area which scored significantly worse than the mean regarding ill fitting doors and windows. Meadow Lane was significantly better than the mean on both counts.

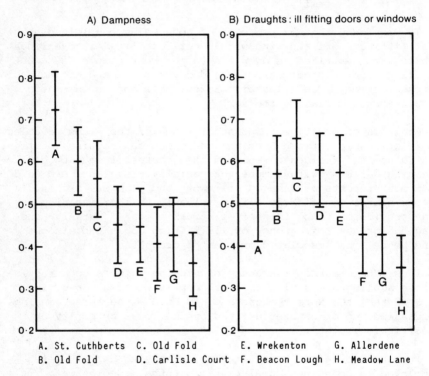

A. St. Cuthberts C. Old Fold   E. Wrekenton   G. Allerdene
B. Old Fold   D. Carlisle Court F. Beacon Lough H. Meadow Lane

Figure 4.1 Housing conditions : mean ridits and 95% confidence
           limits

Environmental defects

Environmental defects were assessed by asking questions about noise and atmospheric pollution. The presence of the latter was gauged simply by asking, 'What do you think about the air around here; does there tend to be a lot of dust, dirt or smoke?' and, 'Does there tend to be a lot of nasty smells?'

Dirty air was most common in St Cuthberts, Nursery Lane and Old Fold. These three housing areas were worse than average on both indicators of environmental pollution. However, the highest frequency of complaints regarding smells were found in Meadow Lane, where 74 per cent of households complained about smells emanating from a local brewery.

The presence of noise was explored using a similar approach to that used to detect the presence of housing defects. Respondents were asked first whether they were bothered by noise, and, if so, what kind of noise, to what extent they were bothered and whether the noise affected the health of household members. Following this a series of questions were asked about noise stemming from specific sources. An ordinal scale was then constructed in the following way:

If bothered by any noise: score 1

If any noise is serious: add 1

If any noise affects health: add 1

If any noise mentioned
        unprompted: add 1

The results of ridit analysis of differences between housing areas regarding scores on the indicator of noise are shown in Figure 4.2. They suggest relatively serious noise problems in St Cuthberts and Nursery Lane which scored well above the sample average. Nursery Lane had a high proportion of noise carried by other people; this noise was caused by rowdy behaviour either outside or inside the building or was simply normal household noise passing through walls that were 'too thin'. St Cuthberts had similar problems but, unlike Nursery Lane, had the additional problem of traffic noise due to its location near the city centre and close to the main railway line.

Dissatisfaction with housing

When directly questioned about their housing conditions people tend to express satisfaction, even when they live in what is clearly sub-standard accommodation. The English House Condition Survey, (DoE, 1978) showed that 87 per cent of households were satisfied (or very satisfied) with their housing. Although degree of satisfaction related, to some extent, to the quality of accommodation, 78 per cent of those who lived in 'unsatisfactory dwellings' were satisfied, along with 68 per cent in dwellings 'lacking amenities', 73 per cent in dwellings 'requiring essential repairs' and 55 per cent in dwellings 'unfit for habitation'.

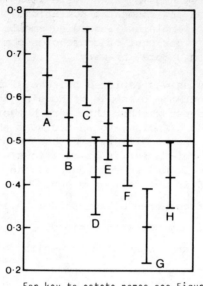

For key to estate names see Figure 4.1

Figure 4.2 Noise : mean ridits and 95% confidence limits

   As has already been noted, the degree of satisfaction varies
with housing type and also with housing tenure. Houses are
more popular than flats, lower floor flats more popular than
those at a higher level, and council tenants are more likely
than average to be unhappy with their housing circumstances.

   The study of housing and health, unlike government surveys
of housing such as the English House Condition Survey, the
National Dwelling and Housing Survey, and the General Household Survey, was restricted to dwellings built for letting by
the local authority. The sample included a higher proportion
of flats and pre 1939 housing than found in the population of
all council housing in Gateshead; higher than normal levels of
dissatisfaction might therefore be expected and this was found
to be the case. Respondents were asked to describe their
attitude to their dwellings on a five point scale ranging from
very satisfied to very dissatisfied - the same as that used by
GHS - and 27 per cent of households claimed to be dissatisfied. Dissatisfaction was not evenly distributed. It was especially high in certain areas, i.e. St Cuthberts (55 per cent),Old

Fold (54 per cent) and Nursery Lane (43 per cent). Thus, the way that people feel about their housing circumstances seemed to vary according to where they lived. In some housing areas a greater proportion of tenants were dissatisfied than satisfied. The three housing areas which were distinctly unpopular all differ in terms of housing form - medium rise flats and maisonettes, high rise flats and 'between war' low rise housing. The similarity between them is that all have been classified by the local authority as 'difficult to let'. Their unpopularity is therefore reflected in the 'letting' difficulties experienced by housing management. In the three 'difficult to let' housing areas 51 per cent of households were dissatisfied; in the other housing areas only 13 per cent of households were dissatisfied.

As Gittus (1976) has suggested, attitudes which people hold towards dwellings in which they live can be complex. These attitudes are not easily measured on a single dimension, and direct questions may in this respect, be inadequate. The housing and health questionnaire included several items which were designed to assess how respondents felt about their living situation. These related to issues connected with the location of dwellings as well as to the dwellings themselves. For instance, respondents were asked:

a) 'Would you say you and your family have a housing problem i.e. is there anything which makes it difficult for you to continue living here?'

b) 'How do you feel about this estate compared to other estates in Gateshead? Would you say it was better than most, worst than most or about average?'

c) 'Have you applied for a transfer since you have been living here?'

d) 'Would you like a transfer?'

In addition, respondents were asked to describe the benefits of living on their particular estate. Dissatisfaction was registered by the 30 per cent of respondents who said there were absolutely no benefits (60 per cent in 'difficult to let' housing areas). On all measures of dissatisfaction there were significant differences between 'difficult to let housing' areas and others.

The individual items were combined to construct a single indicant of housing dissatisfaction by assigning scores of 1 where dissatisfaction was indicated and summing over the items. Cronbach's alpha for this scale was 0.812.

Ridit analysis results, shown in Figure 4.3 suggest a very clear distinction between 'difficult to let' estates and the rest. The 'bad' housing areas - St Cuthberts, Old Fold and Nursery Lane - had significantly higher levels of dissatisfaction than had the 'good' areas. Thus, these housing areas were so unpopular among those who lived in them, that it is not surprising that they are 'difficult to let'. Indeed, as Taylor (1979) suggests, that if they were not 'difficult to live in' then clearly they would not be 'difficult to let'.

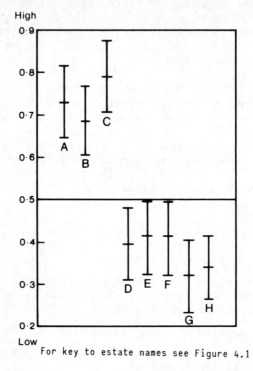

For key to estate names see Figure 4.1

Figure 4.3 Housing dissatisfaction : mean ridits and 95% confidence limits

Regression analysis was used to explore the contribution of certain factors to variance in housing dissatisfaction. The results of this exercise shown in Table 4.5 suggest that housing circumstances play a more important role than personal characteristics; age and sex have non significant effects. The causal model suggested is one which states that people are most likely to be dissatisfied with their housing if they find they have to live in damp houses which they are unable to keep warm, in noisy environments, in 'difficult to let' housing areas; housing area, heating efficacy, noise and dampness are all significant beyond the O.5 level.

Table 4.5
Regression analysis: housing dissatisfaction

		Correlation Coefficient r.	Standardised regression coefficient b.
Age		-.232	-.049
Sex:	1 = male; 2 = female	.025	.018
Health:	1 = good; 2 = fairly good; 3 = not good	.082	.012
Housing area:	1 = 'difficult to let'; O = others	.547	.372*
Housing type:	1 = houses and bungalows O = others	-.184	-.059
Dampness:	O = none to 4 = serious	.374	.094*
Draughts:	O = none to 4 = serious	.267	.037
Heating efficacy:	1 = effective; O = not effective	-.335	-.181*
Dirty air:	1 = yes; O = no	.306	.065
Duration of tenancy:		-.167	.022
Noise:	O = none to 4 = serious	.393	.169*

*R^2 = .427

The insignificant effect of duration of tenancy is surprising in view of Hourihan's (1984) observation that "almost all
studies have shown that length of residence is strongly related to community satisfaction".

RESPONDENTS' PERCEPTIONS OF RELATIONSHIPS BETWEEN HOUSING AND
HEALTH

One aspect of housing and health research which is frequently
neglected concerns the extent to which people themselves
perceive a connection between their health and the dwellings
in which they live. Such perceptions were investigated at
both household and individual levels.

Thirty one per cent of households reported defects which they directly associated with health problems among household members; for the three 'difficult to let' housing areas this was 51 per cent. Thus, over half of the households located in 'difficult to let' housing areas lived in dwellings with structural defects which they considered to be related to ill health.

One of the factors specifically mentioned in the Black Report as a cause of ill health is inadequate heating. As many as 42 per cent of households in the 'housing and health' study said that they had been unable to keep warm during the previous winter. This was a particular problem for those who lived in St Cuthberts, Nursery Lane and Carlisle Court. These housing areas consist of system built flats and maisonettes, which indicates particular problems in heating this kind of dwelling. Fifty six per cent of those unable to keep warm blamed inadequacy of heating systems, while 21 per cent blamed the structure of their dwellings. For 36 per cent of households, inability to keep warm was associated with lack of financial resources necessary to keep heating systems in operation.

The health problems most closely connected with structural defects and inadequate heating were various forms of respiratory disorder. A significant number of respondents also mentioned an association with musculo-skeletal conditions such as rheumatism and arthritis.

In some housing areas the presence of noise can be associated with health problems, especially mental health. Forty four per cent of households were bothered, to some extent, by noise. For 18 per cent of households, noise was a sufficient problem to be associated with poor states of mental health of some household members.

Public sector housing is unique in that access can be achieved through health criteria. Most local authorities have allocation systems which give priority to the 'ill' regarding access to the sector and also to movement within the sector. Such allocation procedures are based on the premise that some houses are more conducive to good health than others, or at least that the health of tenants can be improved by a move to better accommodation. The perceptions of tenants regarding the relationship between their health and their housing conditions may be reflected in applications for housing transfer which give health related reasons. A total of 31 per cent of households of the sample had made official applications for housing transfers; 12 per cent of households had applied

specifically on grounds of ill health. Medical priority
applications were most common among those living in St
Cuthberts, Nursery Lane and Carlisle Court - 23 per cent of
households in these housing areas had made such an applicat-
ion.

The above discussion on perception of relationships between
health and housing deals with data generated at the level of
the household. An alternative approach was to ask individuals
who reported specific health problems whether they thought
that their health could be improved by a change of housing.
This question was asked of all adults who reported respiratory,
nervous or musculo-skeletal conditions. The percentage of
respondents from each housing area with these conditions who
said that their health could be improved by a change of housing
is shown in Table 4.6. These results indicate the presence
of a relatively high degree of perceived housing related ill
health in the three 'difficult to let' housing areas. As
far as nervous and respiratory conditions are concerned there
was no evident difference between flats and some houses. Ill
people who lived in houses in Old Fold saw positive advantages
in moving to better accommodation. For people with musculo-
skeletal conditions the problem appeared to be flats - probably due to difficulty in climbing stairs. However, although
34 per cent of those living in the high rise housing area,
Allerdene, reported musculo-skeletal problems none of these
thought their conditions could be alleviated by transfer to
alternative accommodation.

The evidence suggests that those who live in the worst housing perceive some connection between their housing circumstances and possible ill health. Respondents tended to blame
their housing conditions for poor health of household members
and believed their health could be improved by a move to better housing.

Self-assessments of health and illness

Respondents were asked to rate their (and where relevant their
children's) health over the previous 12 months as: 'good',
'fairly good' or 'not good'. In addition they were asked
whether they had a 'long standing illness' and whether they
had been ill or unwell during the last two weeks. Responses
to those questions did vary between housing areas but the
variation was not always clear cut or consistent. To a large
extent this was due to the confounding effect of age, as
health status tends to decline with increasing years and the
elderly were disproportionately represented in 'good' housing.

97

Table 4.6

Number of respondents reporting various health problems
and number who say problem could be improved by a change of housing

Housing Area	N	Musculo skeletal conditions		Respiratory conditions		Nerves	
		a	b	a	b	a	b
St Cuthberts	84	54	16	61	30	21	16
Old Fold	96	33	7	62	23	41	23
Nursery Lane	67	36	14	53	25	23	20
Carlisle Court	83	34	3	44	7	16	7
Wrekenton	93	52	6	59	6	26	6
Beacon Lough	99	35	4	47	9	17	5
Allerdene	57	21	–	31	4	9	3
Meadow Lane	95	41	5	47	1	18	4
Total	674	306	55	404	105	171	84

Column a : No. reporting a problem
Column b : No. who say problem could be improved by change of housing.

Age was taken into account in two ways, Firstly respondents were asked to rate their health in relation to other people of the same age. A three-point ordinal scale was employed: 'better than others', 'the same as others' and 'worse than others'. Ridit analysis, shown in Figure 4.4 indicates poorer images of health among those who lived in 'difficult to let' housing areas. Those who lived in the prewar slum clearance estate, Old Fold, had significantly worse images of their health, in comparison with people of the same age, than the sample average.

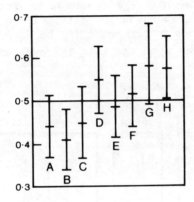

For key to estate names see Figure 4.1

Figure 4.4 Health compared with age group : mean ridits and 95% confidence limits

An alternative way of taking age into consideration is to use it as a control variable. This was done by examining patterns within age sub-groups. However, as the original eight housing areas did not have appropriate age structures to allow age related comparisons between areas, the housing areas were 'collapsed' into two categories; one category contained the three 'difficult to let' estates and the other contained the remaining housing areas. Analysis of housing conditions and residents' opinions suggested that these categories could be

classified as 'bad' and 'good'. The houses in the 'difficult
to let' areas were in the worst physical condition and were
the least popular among tenants, which explains why they are
'difficult to let'.

Figure 4.5 shows results of ridit analysis of the differences between 'difficult to let' housing areas and the rest,
in various age categories, with respect to assessment of
health over the previous 12 months. It is apparent that once
age is taken into consideration the nature of differences
between housing areas becomes clearer. When all ages are
compared there is no significant difference between housing
areas although people in 'difficult to let' housing areas
tended to have poorer images of their health. However, there
are significant differences between housing areas for children
and adults aged between 16 - 24 years old. For all age groups
except for the over 65s those in 'difficult to let' estates
were less healthy than their peers in the more popular estates.
For those over 65 years of age this is reversed.

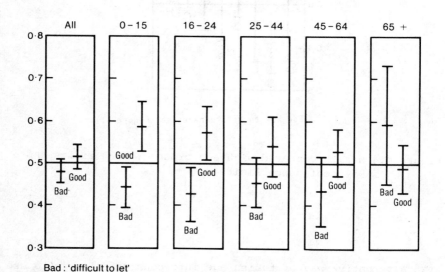

Bad : 'difficult to let'

Good : 'other'

For key to estate names see Figure 4.1

Figure 4.5 Health during last 12 months: mean ridits and 95%
confidence limits

100

Table 4.7 shows the outcome of age controlled analysis of responses to questions about the presence of long standing illness and illness during the previous two weeks (recent illness).

Table 4.7
Illness by CHA controlling for age (percentages)

		Long standing illness	Recent illness	N
0 - 15	Bad	19	42	142
	Good	17	22 **	86
16 - 24	Bad	25	31	78
	Good	17	20	76
25 - 44	Bad	44	35	94
	Good	28 *	18 *	100
45 - 64	Bad	59	41	59
	Good	52	29	136
65 +	Bad	41	41	17
	Good	66	30	114
All	Bad	33	38	390
	Good	39	25	512

Bad : 'difficult to let' $*x^2 > 3.84$; $p < .05$

Good: 'other' $**x^2 > 9.21$; $p < .01$

When all age groups are combined a greater frequency of long standing illness is shown in the 'good' housing areas. However, when the results are broken down it is seen that this is due to the large number of elderly respondents living in 'good' areas. For all age groups except the over 65s, those in 'difficult to let' housing areas were more likely to report long standing illness. Thus, results regarding long standing illness resemble those related to health over the previous 12 months.

For all age groups, people in 'difficult to let' areas were the most likely to have experienced recent illness. Differences were significant for children and for adults aged 25-44 years. However, the 30 per cent of ill people over 65 in the better housing areas contributed considerably to minimising

101

total differences between housing areas. For instance, if the over 65s are excluded from the analysis the total percentages of people in 'difficult to let' areas reporting recent illness does not change while for the others it falls to 23 per cent, thus increasing the difference between housing areas from 13 per cent to 15 per cent.

Conclusions regarding the peculiarity of the results for the over 65s can only be speculative. It may simply be an artifact of the relatively few over 65s in 'difficult to let' housing, but it is more likely to result from the way in which the local authority's letting policies affect the ill elderly. The pattern for recent illness is the same for the elderly as it is for all other groups. If these illnesses are sustained, the probability for transfer to alternative housing increases as ill health itself can be the route to better housing via medical priority policies which give preferential treatment to the ill. Thus, the figures are probably confused because the ill elderly are more likely than their relatively healthy peers to gain access to housing in the 'good' areas, which have long waiting lists. Medical priority movement in this particular authority tends to be out of 'difficult to let' estates. Indeed, ill health can often be the only way to ensure getting out of 'bad' areas into better council housing.

At the bottom end of the age range some disturbing differences were found between housing areas regarding health of children as assessed by the 'mother figure'. Children in 'difficult to let' housing areas were significantly more likely than their peers in the better areas to have experienced recent illness (see Table 4. 7).

Their general health over the previous 12 months was also rated as worse. In addition it was found that children in 'difficult to let' housing areas were more likely to have frequent chesty coughs ($p < .01$) and to have wheezy chests ($p < .01$). These findings cause particular concern in view of the probability that certain related factors are likely to be of less import, e.g. smoking, drinking, occupation and housing history. They suggest that bad housing has a harmful effect from an early age and causes children in 'bad' housing areas to have more health problems than their peers in 'good' areas.

The healthiest group were those aged between 16 and 24 years although there were some significant differences between housing areas. It was found that young adults in 'difficult to let' areas were more likely than those in the 'good' areas to report symptoms of respiratory conditions ($p < .05$) and psychological distress ($p < .05$); they had also been signific-

antly less healthy during the preceding 12 months (p <.0.5).
Similar differences occured in the next age group 25 - 44
where residents in bad areas were significantly more likely to
suffer from long standing or recent illness, to report symptoms of respiratory conditions and psychological distress and
also to have problems with sight (all at significance p <.05).

Although there were clearly some differences between housing
areas, younger adults had the fewest problems concerned with
health; they had grown out of illnesses associated with childhood and had not yet experienced the debilitating effect of
old age. Nevertheless, younger persons living in 'bad' areas
consistently demonstrated poorer self images of health status
than their peers in 'good' areas. The differences between
areas were less likely to have been confounded by medical
priority transfers but in any case these tended to mask the
extent of real differences since they tend to be out of
'difficult to let' housing areas, and into better and more
popular areas.

Differences among younger adults seemed to be particularly
interesting. These were therefore explored further by
examining the intervening effect of social class on differences
between housing areas for all adults aged 16-44 years. Several
studies have suggested a relationship between social class and
health. Some of these were incorporated in evidence presented
by the Black Report (DHSS, 1980) which showed that members of
the lower social classes consistently suffer inferior standards of health compared with those enjoyed by members of the
upper social classes. For instance, a study of the prevalence
of chronic bronchitis among patients aged between 40 and 64
registered with 91 GPs, showed that:

> In terms of GP diagnosis, the percentage
> suffering from chronic bronchitis rose with
> descending class from 6 per cent in Class 1 to
> 26 per cent in Class V. (DHSS, 1980, p.46)

The location of a household in the market is, to a large
extent, dependent upon its location in the class structure.
The households selected for this study share a common location
in a specific housing tenure, a type of tenure designed for
working class consumption. Therefore there is little variation
when households are classified according to the Registrar
General's definitions. In such circumstances, indicators
which reflect levels of working class unemployment and dependence on state financial benefits have potentially more substantive value. A classification based on income dependency was
adopted. This was regarded as a characteristic of households

rather than individuals. Thus, individual members of house-holds were judged to share common class situations based on dependency on state benefits. From this a socio-economic scale was derived. The scale, entitled 'household class' had the following categories:

1. Households containing only pensioners, with no income other than state pension: dependent pensioners

2. Other households which contain only pensioners: non-dependent pensioners

3. Non-pensioner households with no income other than state benefit: dependent

4. Non-pensioner households receiving some state benefits other than child benefits, but also having some alternative sources of income: partially dependent

5. Non-pensioner households not receiving state benefits other than child benefit: non-dependent

Of course, for the 16 - 64 years age group the first two categories are redundant.

Relationships among household class, housing area and per-ceptions of health were explored via log-linear analysis. Log-linear models are similar to statistical procedures such as regression analysis but deal with nominal categories. The units of analysis are cell probabilities; the probability that a randomly selected member of a population has a particular set of characteristics, e.g. the probability of a person from a 'difficult to let' estate, who is a member of the dependent household class describing his health as good.

For log-linear analysis three variables were employed:

A - Housing area: 'difficult to let', others

B - Self assessed health: good, fairly good, not good

C - Household class: dependent, partially dependent, non-dependent

The results of fitting all possible models which describe the relationships between health, housing and household class are shown in Table 4.8. G^2 and significance levels shown in Table 4.8 are indicators of 'goodness of fit'. The closer sign-ificance levels are to 100 per cent the better is the fit with the data. Hence the fully saturated model which includes all variable inter-relationships has a significance of 100 per cent.

Table 4.8
Log-linear analysis of housing area (A), self assessed
health (B) and household class (C)

	Model	G^2	d.f.	sig.
1.	A * B * C	0	0	100%
2.	A * B * + A * C + B * C	0.65	4	95%
3.	A * B + A * C	3.8	8	85%
4.	A * C + B * C	8.6	6	20%
5.	A * B + B * C	115.0	6	Not sig.
6.	A * C + B	19.2	3	Not sig.
7.	A * B + C	125.6	10	Not sig.
8.	B * C + A	130.4	8	Not sig.

The aim of log-linear modelling is to find the most parsimon-
ious model which is the 'best fit'. This turns out to be
model A * B + A * C which states that:

i)   Housing area is inter-related with health

ii) Housing area is inter-related with household class

iii) Household class and health are independent

Thus when household class was controlled, differences
between 'difficult ot let' estates and the rest, regarding
self assessed health, persist. People aged between 16 - 44
years old in 'difficult to let' housing had poorer perception
of their state of health than their peers who lived in better
housing, irrespective of differences in household class.

Musculo-skeletal conditions and restricted activity

Among the 289 adults who claimed to have long standing illness, 27 per cent of the described illnesses were classified
as musculo-skeletal conditions (2). To gain further information about the presence of such conditions and the effect on
ability to lead a normal life questions were asked about the
presence of musculo-skeletal symptoms and also about the ability of respondents to perform certain activities associated
with mobility and normal living patterns (climbing stairs,
bathing, shopping, cutting toe nails, doing heavy housework
and tying a knot in a piece of string).

The ability to perform these activities varied between
housing areas but the variation can be easily explained by
variance in age structure. The areas with most respondents
who reported difficulty or inability to perform tasks were
those which contained the highest proportions of elderly people
- Allerdene, and Meadow Lane. Table 4.9 presents the percentage of people in each age group who found it difficult, or
were unable, to perform each of the tasks. All items are
significantly related to age. Indeed it was found that little
additional explanatory power was achieved by developing models
which included sex, housing area, housing type or household
class. It seems that restriction of activities measured in
this way, is simply a factor of age.

A symptoms approach was used for investigating the presence
of musculo-skeletal problems, and asked the following questions:

 a)   'Do you have difficulty in using your hands?'

 b)   'Do you have trouble with your back and spine?'

 c)   'Do you have difficulty in moving freely and fully?'

 d)   'Do you ever get swollen or painful joints?'

In addition, respondents answering 'yes' to questions b),
c) and d) were also asked:

       'Does it mean you ever have to stay in bed?'

Each 'yes' response was assigned a score of one, then all
scores were summed to provide a cumulative scale ranging from
0 to 7. Cronbach's alpha, for this scale was 0.72.

Validity of this scale was estimated by correlating it with
whether respondents claimed to have a long standing illness or
recent illness classified as musculo-skeletal. Point-biserial
correlations (Guildford, 1965) were calculated; the coefficients were 0.535 for long standing illness and 0.382 for recent
illness. In addition, the correlations between the scale and
each of the activities shown in Table 4.9 were calculated.
The activities were coded:

No difficulty	=	0
Has/would have difficulty	=	1
Cannot do activity	=	2

Correlation coefficients (Pearson's product moment) varied
between 0.239 and 0.472. Therefore all correlations were

Table 4. 9

Difficulty doing/cannot do task by age (percentages)

Age	Climbing stairs ***	Bathing ***	Shopping ***	Tying knot **	Cutting toe-nails ***	Running for bus ***	Heavy housework ***	N
16 - 24	5	3	4	5	3	9	4	149
25 - 44	7	4	10	4	4	19	12	189
45 - 64	23	11	16	9	13	53	28	195
65 +	49	29	32	14	39	78	56	130

** $x^2 > 11.34$; $p < .01$

*** $x^2 > 16.27$; $p < .001$

positive and large enough to suggest that the scale probably
does have some validity.

Figure 4.6   gives results of ridit analysis of the musculo-
skeletal scale. They show that there is no difference between
housing areas, that there is no significant difference between
males and females and that there is a significant relationship
with age. Mean ridits increase considerably within age groups,
although there is some narrowing of differences between the
two older groups.

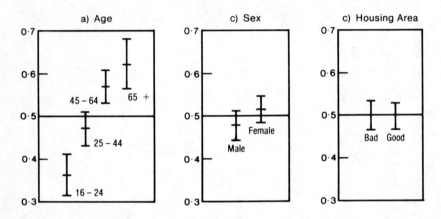

For key to estate names see Figure 4.1

Figure 4.6 Musculo skeletal conditions : mean ridits and 95%
           confidence limits

As one would expect, musculo-skeletal conditions and restricted activity appear to be an outcome of the ageing process.
No evidence of any relationship with housing area or housing
type was found. However, such conditions are likely to be a
major factor in medical priority transfers, especially due to
increasing difficulty which some people experience in climbing
stairs. The result of such transfers move the least mobile
into better housing on 'good' estates, and out of flats into
houses.

Respiratory Conditions

A set of questions designed to elicit presence of symptoms of
respiratory disorders was adapted from a standard questionnaire
often employed by the Medical Research Council (1976). Over
the years substantial evidence has been presented which suggests a causal link between certain housing conditions and
diseases of the chest. In particular, tuberculosis was shown
to be closely connected with overcrowding and lack of basic
amenities. There is litte doubt that a vast improvement in
housing conditions was a major factor in conquering that
particular disease. However, more recently, Morgan and Chenn
(1983) have demonstrated that a link between housing and chest
diseases continues; they showed that children who live in
'urban local authority housing' are more likely than others
to experience illnesses of the respiratory system. Fanning
(1967) compared houses and flats with similar social mixes and
found that general practitioner consultations were more
frequent among flat dwellers of all ages, respiratory problems
being the major reason.

The set of questions which related to symptoms of respiratory
disorders were:

a)   'Do you become breathless or have any pain or fits of
     coughing when you hurry?'

b)   'Do you usually cough first thing in the morning
     (excluding single cough or clearing throat)?'

c)   'Do you usually cough during the day and at night
     (excluding single cough or clearing throat)?'

d)   'Does your chest ever sound wheezy or whistling?'

e)   'Do colds usually go to your chest?

If 'yes' to any:

f)   'Do you have this problem on most days and nights?'

Initial examination of responses regarding these symptoms
revealed a considerable difference between housing areas. On
all the items positive response rates were high among those
who lived in 'difficult to let' housing areas. In addition
there was a tendency for high frequencies of symptoms among
those living in Wrekenton (the 1950s low rise housing estate).

From individual symptom items a cumulative indicator of
respiratory conditions was constructed. Scores of 1 were
assigned to all 'yes' responses, which were then added

together. Thus, the severity of respiratory symptoms was
assumed to be a factor of the number of symptoms present, each
symptom being given equal weight. Cronbach's alpha for this
scale was 0.792.

The validity of the scale was estimated by correlating scores
on the respiratory conditions index with incidences of
respiratory conditions reported as long standing or recent
illness. Point-biserial correlations (Guildford, 1965) were
calculated; these were 0.41 for respiratory conditions related
to long standing illness, and 0.25 for respiratory conditions
during the previous two weeks. Respondents were also asked
whether they had ever had bronchitis, pleurisy or pneumonia;
point-biserial correlations for these items with the respiratory conditions index were 0.47, 0.29 and 0.27 respectively.
Thus correlations with each of the five items were not large,
but all were in the correct direction and large enough to
suggest that the scale does have some validity.

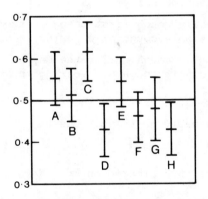

For key to estate names see Figure 4.1

Figure 4.7 Respiratory conditions : mean ridits and 95%
confidence limits

110

Results of ridit analysis of differences between housing areas, are shown in Figure 4.7. They support the tentative conclusions drawn from the preliminary analysis of the distribution of individual symptoms. Mean scores are significantly higher than the sample average in Nursery Lane and they are relatively high in St Cuthberts, Old Fold and Wrekenton. Rates are lower than average in Carlisle Court and Meadow Lane. On this evidence, respiratory conditions do not appear to be related to housing type. The four housing areas which are made up of houses have varying mean scores; Old Fold and Wrekenton score above the mean while Beacon Lough and Meadow Lane score below. There is also variation between the two housing areas which consist of medium rise dwellings; scores are high in St Cuthberts but low in Carlisle Court and these two housing areas are significantly different from each other. There are also significant differences between the two high rise housing areas, with high scores in Nursery Lane and low scores in Allerdene, despite the presence of large numbers of elderly in the latter. Therefore there is no evident pattern which suggests a relationship between respiratory conditions and housing type.

To explore relationships in the data further, analysis of variance techniques were employed with five independent variables: housing area, housing type, household class, smoking and experience of working in unhealthy environments; in addition, age was included as a covariate. All of these factors have at some time been related to presence of respiratory disorders (see Gibson, 1981).

The five variables were classified as follows:

Housing area :   'difficult to let'; others

Housing type :   houses and bungalows; low to medium rise flats and maisonettes; high rise dwellings (i.e. dwellings located in blocks of over eight storeys).

Housing class: households with no income other than state benefit (state dependent); households receiving some state benefits other than child benefit but also having some alternative source of income (partially dependent); households receiving no state benefits other than child benefit (non-dependent).

Smoking   :   smoker; ex-smoker; passive smoker (non smoker but other members of the household smoke); non smoker (no members of the household smoke.

Worked in   :   classified from response to the question
unhealthy   'Have you ever worked in what you consi-
environment   dered to be an unhealthy environment?'
                        - i.e. yes; no.

Figure 4.8 shows that there are clear and constant differences between housing areas for all age groups apart from the
over 65s. This suggests an interaction between age and housing area which, potentially, could be problematic. This problem was solved by excluding the over 65s from multi-variate
analysis which meant that interaction between age and housing
area was controlled for simply by omitting the sub group
responsible for that interaction.

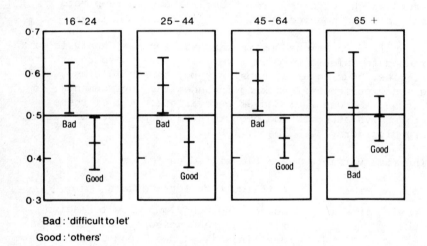

Bad : 'difficult to let'
Good : 'others'

For key to estate names see Figure 4.1

Figure 4.8 Respiratory conditions by age and housing area :
       mean ridits and 95% confidence limits

Conventional methods of analysis of variance tend to be unsuitable for analysis of survey results. They are appropriate
for experimental designs which have equal, or at least propor-
tionate, cell frequencies. Survey data seldom have the neat
proportionality of experimental designs which means that main
effects and interactions are not additive; they tend to be

112

entangled amongst each other, which makes results difficult to interpret. Schuessler (1972) suggests that the way round this problem is to use the 'method of fitted constants' which is in effect a form of analysis of variance. The fitting of constants requires an assumption that there is no interaction in the model; in this case, first order interactions were non-significant (p =<.13) and higher order interactions could not be calculated due to the presence of empty cells.

Table 4.10 gives the results of fitting constants for the main effects. These suggest that smoking had the most significant effect on respiratory conditions, but the effects of housing area and experience of working in unhealthy environments were also significant. When these factors were taken into consideration neither household class nor housing type were significantly related to respiratory conditions.

Table 4.10

Fitted constants - analysis of covariance

	Sum of Squares	d.f.	F	Significance of F
Within cells	3138	395	-	-
Regression	58	1	7.4	.007
Constant	116	1	14.6	.000
Household class	13	2	0.8	.454
Smoking	373	3	15.7	.000
Housing Type	18	2	1.1	.331
Housing Area	52	1	6.5	.011
Worked in unhealthy environment	190	1	23.9	.000

The relationships between these variables were further explored by way of a multiple classification analysis, which examines patterns of relationships between independent and dependent variables. It is a useful technique for displaying analysis of variance results, and shows the net effect on each variable when differences in other factors are controlled for.

Column (a) in Table 4.11 gives the deviation from the mean of the various categories of each independent variable; column (b) gives a value of eta, - equivalent to a correlation co-

Table 4.11

Multiple classification analysis

		(a) Deviations from mean - unadjusted	(b) eta	(c) Deviations from mean - adjusted for independent and co-variates	(d) beta
Household Class	Dependent	0.28		- 0.14	
	Partially dependent	0.40		0.26	
	Non-dependent	- 0.47	0.13	- 0.05	0.05
Smoking	Non smoker	- 1.56		- 1.48	
	Passive smoker	- 1.43		- 0.92	
	Ex-smoker	- 0.39		- 0.65	
	Smoker	0.92	0.34	0.80	0.29
Dwelling Type	Houses	- 0.31		- 0.10	
	Low to medium rise flats	- 0.00		- 0.03	
	High rise flats	1.44	0.17	0.54	0.06
Housing Area	'Difficult to let' (Bad)	0.68		0.52	
	Other (Good)	- 0.43	0.17	- 0.34	0.13
Worked in unhealthy environment	No	- 0.58		- 0.46	
	Yes	1.09	0.25	0.86	0.20

$R^2 = 0.208$

114

efficient - which indicates the relation of each single fact-
or with scores on the respiratory conditions index. From
column (a) it can be observed that:

(i)   Respondents from partially dependent households had
      higher levels of respiratory conditions than those
      from dependent households who in turn scored higher
      than members of non-dependent households.

(ii) There are progressively higher scores on the smoking
      variable with non smokers having the least respiratory
      problems and smokers the most.

(iii) Respondents who lived in houses had less severe respir-
      atory conditions than those who lived in low to medium
      rise flats who in turn were healthier than residents of
      high rise blocks.

(iv) Those who lived in 'difficult to let' housing areas had
      higher levels of respiratory conditions than the rest.

(v)   Those who had worked in unhealthy environments were
      more likely to have respiratory problems than those
      who had not.

Column (c) in Table 4.11 gives deviations from the mean for
each category of each variable when the effect of the other
independent variables and the covariate (age) are taken into
consideration. Column (d) gives a beta coefficient which
gives the unique effect of each independent variable - i.e.
the relationship with the respiratory conditions index when
the variance which is shared with the other variates and covariates is removed. Thus, column (d) shows that when the
effect of other independent and covariates are adjusted, the
effects of household class and dwelling type are virtually
removed.

From this model it is concluded that respiratory conditions
are a factor of smoking habits, location in 'bad' housing
areas and experience of employment in unhealthy environments.
In terms of housing, respiratory conditions are associated
with dwelling location rather than dwelling type.

Several factors have traditionally been associated with
disorders of the respiratory system. On the evidence presented here smoking is the most important factor which supports
findings made frequently in other research (e.g. Lambert and
Reid, 1970; Hawthorne and Fry, 1978; Dean et al., 1978). It
was found that those who currently smoked cigarettes had the
highest level of respiratory conditions, followed by ex-
smokers and then passive smokers; the most healthy individuals
in this sense, were those who had never smoked and who lived in

non-smoking households. In this context it was disturbing to note that the Health Education Council's antismoking campaign seems to be having limited impact. As many as 201 respondents (31 per cent of adults) were of the opinion either that smoking did not affect health or that it depended on the amount smoked. These opinions were expressed by 38 per cent of all smokers.

High rates of chest disorders are commonly found in industrial environments (Girt, 1972). Those who are employed in unhealthy environments are especially vulnerable (Gibson, 1981). Only limited information on employment history was collected but insight was gained from a question regarding whether the respondents had ever worked in an environment which they thought was bad for their health. This simple variable accounted for 11 per cent of the variance in respiratory conditions.

The principal purpose of the survey was to examine the hypothesis that poor housing is related to poor health, respiratory conditions being one of the health factors of specific interest. The evidence found suggests that people who live in housing areas which include most of the very worst housing i.e. 'difficult to let' estates, are more likely to report symptoms of respiratory disorders than those who live in the better housing areas.

The index of respiratory conditions was applied to adults only, but 'mother figures' were asked two questions which were similar to those directed to adults. These were:

a)   'Do any of your children tend to have frequent chesty coughs?'

b)   'Do any of your children's chests ever sound wheezy or whistling?'

Forty seven per cent of children living in 'difficult to let' housing areas were said to have frequent chesty coughs; for children living in the remaining housing areas the rate was 27 per cent. In 'difficult to let' housing areas 40 per cent of children had wheezy or whistling chests, as opposed to 20 per cent in other housing areas. For both items the difference between housing areas was statistically significant ($p < .01$). Put another way, the rates suggest, all other factors being equal, that 20 per cent of children in 'difficult to let' estates have chesty coughs or wheezy chests because they live in 'bad' housing.

Psychological Distress

A number of research studies have suggested an association between the type of dwellings which people occupy and their states of mental health. The usual conclusion is that flat dwellers are more likely than those who live in houses to have experienced various forms of mental disorder, and that vulnerability increases according to the height of dwelling (e.g. Fanning,1967; Richman,1974; Hannay, 1979). Littlewood and Tinker (1981) in their follow up study of families that had moved out of high rise dwellings, found that fewer symptoms of depression were reported after the move.

As in the case of other health factors, the effect of housing on mental health can be difficult to establish. Psychological states have been associated with several factors which may themselves be correlated with housing circumstances, such as class, income, sex and physical health.

Brown and Harris (1978) and Turner and Noh (1983) found that symptoms of depression are to a large extent the result of class experiences. Low status groups are particularly vulnerable.

Women are generally found to be more susceptible to mental disorders than men (e.g. Aneshensel et al.,1981; Kessler and McCrae,1981; Cleary and Mechanic,1983). An extensive review of the literature was undertaken by Dohrenwend and Dohrenwend (1976) who found that in 28 out of 32 studies of neurosis and 18 out of 24 studies of manic-depression females had higher rates than men. It has been proposed that higher rates among women, in self report studies, result from the greater relunctance of men to admit to 'unpleasurable feelings and sensations' (Phillips and Segal, 1969). However, Clancy and Grove(1974) examined this hypothesis and concluded that differences between men and women were not an artifact of response bias.

Kessler and Mechanic (1978), Murray et al (1982) and Hannay (1979) all observed significant correlations, in self report studies, between physical health and mental health. However, these kinds of associations present problems regarding identification of causality. The studies mentioned appear to treat poor physical health as a cause of poor mental health, when it would be equally logical to suggest that cause and effect operate in the opposite direction; people may have poor perceptions about their health because they are psychologically distressed. It seems possible that causal connections are circular; poor health may cause psychological distress which causes poor health, and so on.

The extent of psychological distress was estimated by posing questions derived from Brown and Harris (1978) and Townsend (1979), about the presence of symptoms, viz:

1) 'Are you affected by

    a) depression or weeping so that you can't face your work or mix with people?

    b) being unable to concentrate?

    c) sleeping badly

    d) feeling that it's too much effort to do anything?

    e) feeling helpless and overwhelmed?

    f) loss of appetite?'

2) 'Do you have trouble with your nerves?

'Yes' responses proved to be considerably more frequent among people who lived in the 'difficult to let' housing areas. There was no relationship with dwelling type. This suggested that psychological distress was a factor connected with the location of a dwelling, rather than whether that dwelling was a flat or a house.

Responses to the set of symptoms questions were used to construct an index of psychological distress by summing all 'yes' responses. Cronbach's alpha for the scale was 0.827. It was not possible to check the validity of the scale because there were too few instances of long standing or recent illness which could be classified as mental disorders for them to be incorporated as a check on construct validity.

Figure 4.9. shows the ridit analysis of variations between housing areas regarding scores on the psychological distress index. St Cuthberts, Nursery Lane and Old Fold all have mean ridits which are above the sample average. For Old Fold and Nursery Lane these differences are significant. All of the 'good' housing areas have mean ridits which are below the sample average; for Allerdene and Meadow Lane the difference is significant.

Figure 4.9. suggests that the housing areas can be grouped into three distinct categories each of which contains a mixture of housing types.

    a) *High distress areas* - St Cuthberts, Old Fold and Nursery Lane, all 'difficult to let' housing areas: one area is low to medium rise dwellings, one is high rise dwellings

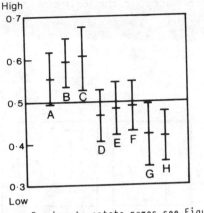

For key to estate names see Figure 4.1

Figure 4.9 Psychological distress : mean ridits and 95%
confidence limits

and one is low rise, traditionally built houses.

b) *Intermediate areas* - Carlisle Court, Wrekenton and
Beacon Lough: two areas of houses and one of medium
rise, system built flats.

c) *Low distress areas* - Meadow Lane and Allerdene: one
area of houses and one area of high rise flats.

Clearly there is some form of interaction between housing
type and housing location e.g. high rise flats in 'difficult
to let' housing areas are associated with high distress while
the same type of dwelling located in 'good' areas is
associated with low distress.

When differences between dwelling type were examined it was
found that high rise flats were associated with the highest
levels of distress, followed by low to medium rise dwellings
with the lowest level of psychological distress found among
occupants of housing. However, differences were small and not
statistically significant.

As in the case of health over the previous 12 months, long standing illness, recent illness and respiratory conditions, there was evidence of pronounced interaction between housing area and age. The results of the relevant ridit analysis are shown in Figure 4.10.

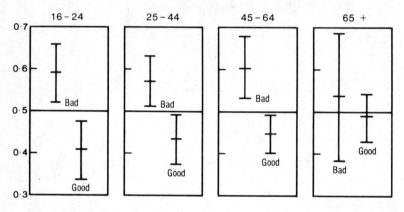

Bad : 'difficult to let'
Good : 'others'

For key to estate names see Figure 4.1

Figure 4.10 Psychological distress by age and housing area :
mean ridits and 95% confidence limits

Again, a pattern may be observed where there is a significant difference between housing areas for all age groups except for the over 65s. In every age group, with the exception of the elderly, people who lived in 'difficult to let' housing were more distressed than their peers living in 'good' housing areas. For elderly respondents there was no difference between housing areas. Once again the most likely explanation relates to the effect of transfer policies which move the ill elderly out of the 'bad' areas and into the 'good' areas.

A multivariate approach was employed to explore further the network of relationships between housing area, housing type and psychological distress. The aim was to examine the effects of housing type and housing area upon psychological distress when the intervening effects of age, sex, physical health and household class were taken into consideration. This was basically an analysis of covariance problem. As was the case with analysis of respiratory conditions, traditional methods were invalidated due to unequal and disproportionate cell frequencies. In addition there was a further difficulty, as preliminary analysis had suggested interaction between the independent variables. Thus the unique sum of squares was calculated, that is, the amount of variance which is unique to the independent variables and also the interaction between them.

The independent variables were:

Housing area: 'difficult to let'; others

Housing type: houses, bungalows; low to medium rise houses and flats; high rise flats.

The intervening variables were:

Age

Household class: dependent = 1; partially dependent = 2; non dependent = 3

Sex   :   male = 1; female = 2

Self assessed :   very good = 1; fairly good = 2; health   not good = 3

As with the health indicators analysed earlier, interaction between housing area and age was controlled by excluding the elderly from the analysis.

Table 4.12

Analysis by weighted mean squares with age,
sex, health and household class as intervening variables:
psychological distress

	F-ratio	Standardised regression co-efficient	Significance
Age		.047	.249
Health		.429	<.001
Sex		.185	<.001
Household class		- .015	.703
Regression	42.1		<.001
Constant	5.7		.017
Housing type	0.3		.740
Housing Area	22.17		<.001
Interaction	4.19		.016

The outcome of analysis of covariance is shown in Table 4.12. The results give confirmation of the presence of interaction between housing type and housing area, and also of the significant effect of housing area. Housing type on its own is not related to psychological distress. Thus, on this evidence, psychological distress is associated with where a person lives but not by the type of dwelling which he or she occupies.

The presence of interaction is, to a large extent, accounted for by the differences between the two housing areas consisting only of high rise flats. People living in Nursery Lane had the highest mean levels of psychological distress, while those who lived in the same dwelling type in Allerdene were among the least distressed. Thus, high rise flat dwellers in one location were the most psychologically distressed while those in another location showed low levels of distress.

At this point it is worth considering differences between the two high rise housing areas. The sociodemographic composition of each is determined, to a large extent, by the local authority's policy of not letting high rise dwellings to families with children. The result of this is that high rise flats in 'difficult to let' areas tend to be let to single or divorced people or to young married couples. Occupants of these flats tend to see their housing circumstances as temporary; they may be saving for a mortgage or, alternatively, hope for housing transfers if and when they have children. Examination of lettings records of the local authority revealed that in Nursery Lane, 27 per cent of dwellings changed hands over a six month period; 72 per cent of these dwellings were let to people from the council housing waiting list who were classified as 'living-in'. Over a two year period 36 tenants were transferred out for 'medical' reasons and in the same period 31 per cent of dwellings had remained unoccupied for periods exceeding three months.

In many ways Allerdene is the complete opposite to Nursery Lane. Turnover of dwellings over a six months period, was seven per cent. Thirty seven per cent of the re-lets went to elderly persons on the waiting list and 25 per cent went to elderly persons transferring from other council accommodation. Over a two year period only one person was transferred out through medical priority procedures; six were transferred in. Respondents on these estates tended to have been rehoused from private tenancies or owner occupation in inner city areas or transferred from council housing following dispersal of nuclear family units. They tended to be satisfied with their housing circumstances, considered them to be permanent and had no desire to move out.

Nursery Lane is a typical example of inner city, high rise
housing. Such estates emerged as a response to problems
created by overcrowding in inner cities. However, they proved
to be no solution to many of the social problems associated
with life in inner cities (poverty, unemployment, delinquency)
and tended to create new problems. They are unpopular, tend
to have high turnovers and dwellings are 'difficult to let'.
The result is that these estates contain many empty and
boarded up properties and become 'sump' estates which event-
ually contain multiple social problems.

Allerdene is an example of high rise accommodation which has
the function of moving people out of the inner cities. High
rise flats like this are located in pleasant housing areas in
the suburbs, away from the problems and pollution of the inner
city. This type of accommodation is integrated with low rise,
good quality housing with easy access to open countryside and
views which overlook green fields, rather than factories.
Their location means that they have far fewer problems with
noise than similar dwellings located close to city centres.

The housing type associated with lowest levels of psychological distress was 'houses and bungalows'. Yet even among
these there were distinct variations. The housing area with
the second highest level of psychological distress, Old Fold,
consists totally of houses and bungalows, which suggests that
there are problems associated with houses in some housing
areas or that psychological distress is not simply a factor
of living in a flat.

The regression coefficients shown in Table 4.12 allow
comparison between the effects of the intervening variables.
Physical health is the most important of these, but as suggested above there are doubts about the causal direction of the
relationship between self assessed health and mental health.

Sex is significantly related to psychological distress (b =
.185;   p <.001). Women had higher levels of psychological
distress than men; a finding which is consistent with those
of most studies of mental health; however, as might be
expected, unemployed men reported a higher level of 'trouble
with nerves' than those in gainful employment (p <.02).
Household class and age, on their own, were not significantly
related to psychological distress.

CONCLUSION

The analysis of survey results began by looking at differences
in housing conditions and degrees of satisfaction expressed
by the occupants of council housing. Distinct variations were
found. People living in 'difficult to let' housing areas were
the most likely to report housing and environmental defects
and were correspondingly the most dissatisfied with their
housing circumstances. 'Difficult to let' housing areas were
clearly unpopular among those who lived in them. Dissatisfaction is determined by the way in which an individual percei-
ves certain characteristics of a dwelling and the area in
which it is located. The evidence drawn from this survey
suggests that poor conditions can be found in various types
of dwellings, and that dissatisfaction is determined more by
the location of a dwelling than by the dwelling type or the
presence of structural defects.

When differences between housing areas regarding self assessed health were examined, it was found that the same patterns
emerged as regards differences in housing conditions and housing circumstances. On all indicators, people living in
'difficult to let' housing areas reported more illness and
inferior health status than did people living in the other
housing areas. Consistent differences between housing areas
were found which could be explained more by the location of a
dwelling than by dwelling type.

The sample included three housing areas defined by the local
authority as 'difficult to let' estates. These estates are
different from each other in that they consist of different
types of housing; St Cuthberts is mostly low to medium rise,
system built flats and maisonettes; Old Fold is traditionally
built low rise housing; Nursery Lane is system built, high
rise accommodation. It was found that people living in these
housing areas were similar on most health indicators. They
were the group most likely to identify connections between
ill health among household members and bad housing conditions.
They were likely to have poorer perceptions of their own
health, and report greater frequencies of long standing
and recent illness than those who lived in the 'good' housing
areas. People who lived in 'difficult to let' housing areas
reported greater frequencies of respiratory symptoms and
symptoms of psychological distress than those who lived in
'good' areas; correspondingly, they scored significantly higher on indices of respiratory conditions and psychological
distress, which were derived from the individual symptoms.

When examining the effects of housing type it was generally found that people who lived in houses were healthier than those who lived in flats, and that people who lived in low to medium rise blocks of flats were healthier than those who lived in high rise blocks. However, differences between housing types which were statistically significant were not found. This was due to differences between similar dwelling types which could be explained by whether or not they were located in 'difficult to let' housing areas.

Peet (1975) suggests that cities can be described as complexes of 'hierarchical living spaces'. Some social environments are more desirable and consequently more sought after than others. The social environment in which an individual is located is crucial because it determines his life chances through a network of services, information and connections. An individual's life chances will vary according to his ability to exploit what Peet describes as the 'daily-life environment'. But, the extent to which an environment can be exploited depends on mobility, the ability to move into more advantageous living spaces. The degree of mobility is dependent on the ability to exercise bargaining power in housing markets. Absence of power results in location at the lower end of the housing hierarchy in the least desirable and least advantageous housing spaces.

Hierarchy of living space clearly exists in the local authority housing sector. Some housing estates are more sought after than others, with correspondingly more applications for houses and longer waiting lists. The simplest level of hierarchical ranking is the classification of certain housing areas as 'difficult to let'. Although there tend to be long waiting lists for council property, housing departments inevitably have difficulty in persuading prospective tenants to accept accommodation in some areas. Consequently only those without bargaining power actually agree to live in these areas. The majority of lettings regarding all Gateshead 'difficult to let' estates are to people on the waiting list who are classified as 'living in' - generally young couples living with one of their nuclear families. Those not let to this category tend to be let to the 'homeless' or to people who have moved from 'out of the borough'. Thus, location in 'difficult to let' housing areas is not so much a result of "the grading of prospective tenants" (Ineicher, 1983) but more usually the absence of choice among particular groups of people. The absence of choice is a result of housing circumstances which do not permit prospective tenants the luxury of awaiting better offers.

Once tenants have entered the 'difficult to let' housing
strata they have great difficulty leaving it unless they acqu-
ire sufficient funds to buy into the private sector or become
sufficiently ill to warrant medical priority transfer. Most
of them do want to move out. Of those households located in
'difficult to let' housing areas 78 per cent expressed a desire
to move out of their current accommodation, of which only
nine per cent would accept a dwelling located on the same
estate. Fifty three per cent of households had already submitted official applications to the local authority's housing
department. Those who are unable to move out tend to feel
trapped in their current housing circumstances, with which
they are distinctly dissatisfied, and are vulnerable to illness and psychological distress.

The 1980 Housing Act gave sitting tenants the 'right to
buy' their council housing, with discounts based upon the
length of occupancy. This policy gives undeniable benefit to
tenants fortunate enough to occupy a desirable dwelling and
sufficient income to exercise their 'right to buy'. However,
purchases have been shown to be selective (Forrest, 1982), and
sales have been concentrated in locations which are considered
to be at the upper end of the council housing hierarchy - the
'good' council housing.

Of the 2,939 applications to purchase council houses under
the terms of the 1980 Act that were examined, only two per
cent related to dwellings which were classified via cluster
analysis in the worst housing (Clusters 1 and 2) although these
clusters accounted for 12 per cent of all dwellings. Ninety
three per cent of applications related to dwellings contained
in two of the clusters of 'good' housing.

Council house sales have contributed towards worsening the
circumstances of those who live in 'difficult to let' housing.
They cause increased ghettoisation of some housing areas.
The selective nature of sales removes the best local authority
stock into the private sector and adversely affects opportunities for transfers out of the worst housing. Medical priority transfer systems have served to counter some of the health
effects of bad housing. Their role is to afford opportunities
for ill council tenants to move into environments which are
more conducive to good health. The 'right to buy' decreases
the supply of good housing, thus condemning the ill and the
psychologically distressed to longer periods in housing
circumstances which may be contributing towards, or even
causing, their condition.

NOTES

(1)   Several papers concerned with the debate concerning
        measurement and choice of statistical methods are
        included in Bernhardt Lieberman (ed.) *Contemporary
        Problems in Social Statistics: a book of readings
        for the behavioural sciences,* Oxford University
        Press, New York, 1971.

(2)   Illnesses were classified according to the
        *International classification of health problems in
        primary care,* (1979).

5 Policy implications

INTRODUCTION

> ... the solution of the housing problem will
> confer much more good on the community than
> the complete fulfilment of the National Health
> Service Act. (MOH for Gateshead, 1948)

It is perfectly clear that both the housing conditions and
the health of people in the United Kingdom in the 1980s are
much better than they were forty years ago. However, the
burden of the Black Report (1980) is that relative inequalities in health have not changed. Clearly the Black Report is
informed by a concept of 'relative health' which derives explicitly from the concept of relative poverty. The clearest
assertion of egalitarianism in the social policy of the
United Kingdom is that contained in the 1946 National Health
Service Act. This chapter is written with the underlying
assumption that that egalitarianism remains the predominant
social attitude towards health policy, an assumption which
receives refreshing support from the *British Social Attitudes
Survey*, (1984, Chapter 4), however little it may accord with
the intentions and practices of the present government.
However, the following discussion will assume that this is
not the dominant view. Thus, the policy implications of that
which has gone before will be outlined in relation to an overall policy objective which can be stated as that of bringing

the health of the less healthy up to the health level of the most healthy.

These policy implications will be discussed under four headings. These are: action with regard to the existing housing stock; action with regard to the organisation of the health services in relation to housing issues; action with regard to the design, construction and location of housing in the future; and, finally, a discussion of policy for research and policy and research.

Action with regard to the existing housing stock

In the 1930s the future Lord Simon of Wythenshawe wrote a book called *How to abolish the slums* (1929). That question is still faced today, although the locale of the slums is now very different. There is in this country a legislative and administrative system which is concerned with the quality control of the overall housing stock through the elimination of deficient, old private housing. The continued appropriateness of that system has been questioned since the mid 1960s, for example by Dennis (1970, 1972). By now it can be said to have achieved its objectives; it has eradicated the appalling mess that was imposed in housing terms on the urban population of the United Kingdom in the first half of the nineteenth century. As will be seen, one part of the system, the direct input of medical expertise and status through the MOH, has to all intents and purposes, been abolished. Since the mid 1960s part of that system, and in particular the environmental health officer, has been transferred to a new type of role, namely, that of conserving rather than eradicating older housing. The community physician, whose function is a remnant of that of the MOH, has been reduced to the role of rationing cases of 'medical priority' for rehousing, or more often transfer, in relation to the public sector stock.

There is one clear implication of the research and analysis reported in this book. It is that the 'slums' which matter today are those located in the public sector stock. It is perfectly clear in Gateshead that dwellings which were being considered for clearance at the time that St Cuthberts Village was built, will outlast that estate by many years. Those dwellings may have major problems of structural repair which was outside the scope of the survey reported here, but they are potentially a useful part of the housing stock from which provision will be made for the foreseeable future. The 'bad' areas in the public sector are not.

This raised three sets of problems. How are these 'bad areas' to be managed while they are as they are? What is an appropriate strategy for dealing with them? How is such a strategy to be converted into a system for its implementation? At present the first set of problems are conceived of in terms of 'housing management'. The first central recognition of the issue was by the Housing Development Directorate in its studies of 'difficult to let' estates (DoE, 1980b, 1980c, 1980d). The recognition was not an original one. James Tucker's pioneering *Honourable Estates* (1966) had clearly identified the degree of social segregation existing within the council housing system and the issue had been returned to in the 1970s (e.g. Damer, 1976) and by almost all of the Home Office sponsored Community Development Projects. These authors, together with the 1980 DoE studies, all recognised the structural origins (in a literal sense) of the difficulties posed by this stock. It is therefore unfortunate that the present course of policy sponsored by the Department of Environment through its 'Priority estates' programme (1981) seems concerned with managing rather than eradicating the problem.

In an article in *Housing Review* (Sept./Oct. 1981) which reported on a discussion of the document describing the 'Priority estates' project, one of the authors of that report was quoted as saying that it was time to abandon the 'edifice based approach'; that one ought to equate a housing estate with a hospital and judge it not just in terms of the building but in relation to its 'staff' of residents and managers. Clearly there are instances where managerial solutions are appropriate. The frequently quoted example of the Springwell estate in Gateshead is one where a 'difficult to let' estate has been turned round by intensive housing management. However, in Springwell the problem was managerial in origin, relating to the allocation of a particular set of conventional dwellings to a residue of large families at the end of a slum clearance programme. In an estate where the 'edifices' were acceptable, a management solution has proved effective. In contrast, in St Cuthberts Village, intensive management has not resolved the difficulties, even in managerial terms.

It is necessary to identify the nature of the problem of 'difficult to let' estates in management terms. The Housing Development Directorate have pointed out, quite rightly, that many of these are not 'difficult to let' but just difficult to let to anybody who has any choice in the matter, and therefore:

> ... progressively accumulate a concentration of
> families who are on low incomes, who are unemployed

or who have other related social problems.
This tendency for families who are less able
to cope to end up in housing which is in least
demand we have called 'social polarization'.
(DoE, 1980b, p.1)

The real problems emerge when the estates are 'difficult to
let' as well. The housing manager is acutely concerned about
'voids', about long term empty dwellings producing no rental
income and incurring increased repair and maintenance expenditure as a consequence of vandalism and the inevitable deter-
ioration of non occupation. The high incidence of 'voids'
in non traditionally built estates, even at a time of severe
housing shortage and increasing waiting lists, is of particular
interest. Tenants are 'voting with their feet', refusing to
accept allocations to these areas and abandoning them through
transfer and re-entry into the remaining private sector,
although as Taylor (1979) has indicated, they are 'difficult
to get out of'. What then is to be done with this stock?

Some is being sold into the private sector either as job
lots for conversion into 'town houses' (local North East
examples of this include the conversion of maisonettes in
Newcastle by a commercial building firm or the sale of
very cheap flats to individuals in 'difficult to let' areas of
Washington New Town). In some cases, ownership and responsib-
ility has been transferred to the tenants by a process of
conversion to tenant cooperatives. In others, property has
been demolished or is intended for demolition. In December
1984 the Housing Committee of Gateshead Metropolitan
Borough Council decided to demolish a large part of St
Cuthberts Village and four out of five 'difficult to let'
high rise blocks at Nursery Lane. The remaining block will be
upgraded by considerable capital investment and converted for
use by single persons. In discussion at the Housing Committee there was clear recognition that the partial demolition
of St Cuthberts was an interim measure, that the estate
as a whole did not have a long term future, but that the
housing shortage in the borough was so severe that it could
not be completely demolished at the present time. (1)

The slums dealt with up to and including the 1957 Housing Act
(the legislation currently in force), have been old dwellings
in the private sector. Privately rented, 'unfit' dwellings
are acquired at site value, that is, in effect, 'confiscated'.
Owner occupiers receive an owner occupier's supplement which
gives them the market value of their dwelling, even if it is
classified unfit. Indeed, the increasing importance of
owner occupation as a tenure in potential clearance areas and
the consequent compensation costs is yet one more factor

operating against clearance as a contemporary policy. The
'confiscation' of privately rented dwellings is in fact quite
justifiable in almost any political terms. The dwellings
concerned were built between 80 and 100 years ago and their
original cost has long ago been written off. Although the
Inland Revenue does not allow depreciation against rental
income, the effect of inflation can be argued to be broadly
the same in practice. If this view is held, privately rented
slums can quite properly be treated as totally depreciated
assets which have no intrinsic worth. Clearly, there are
political reasons for not treating owner occupiers in the same
way and since the 1980 Housing Act, absentee landlords in
clearance areas have been able to obtain 'standard' improvements grants which have ensured that unfit dwellings can be
converted into 'fit' dwellings which then attract full market
value compensation.

The picture with regard to contemporary public sector slums
is much more complex. In the first place the role of
environmental health officers in regulating the quality of
public sector stock is not clear. In principle they can
employ all their powers of notice and orders, but they are
actually employees of the landlords concerned and in many
authorities have been, either explicitly or implicitly,
precluded from a role with regard to the public sector. In
Gateshead, for example, which is by no means a 'bad practitioner' in this regard, environmental health officers were first
permitted to have a role in relation to council housing in
1984.

Historically, the clearance process has been connected with
the demonstration of differential health outcomes and the
achievement of better health through rehousing. However, the
absence of any such clearance process with respect to
contemporary public sector slums has meant that the health
inadequacies of 'mass housing' have not yet been revealed.
Indeed, the financial difficulties associated with the clearance of dwellings which have not been depreciated in financial
terms are very considerable. Typically, public sector housing
finance is so constructed that the initial capital costs are
written off over a 60 year period. Given the existence of the
pooled Housing Revenue Account and consequent rent pooling,
any connection between the historic cost of any particular
part of public sector stock and the actual rents charged for
that stock is tenuous but, in principle, loans cover a 60 year
period. If an English local authority is 'out of subsidy',
i.e. no longer in receipt of general exchequer subsidies to
its Housing Revenue Account as a consequence of the operation
of the 1980 Housing Act, the central government will not
allocate resources to enable the writing off of the debt

charge. Indeed while it has only recently been agreed that an
'in subsidy' authority can continue to receive subsidies for
cleared stock no special provision is made for the costs of
clearance. Gateshead is 'out of subsidy' and Gateshead's
council tenants and ratepayers will therefore continue to pay
debt charges on Nursery Lane and St Cuthberts Village for more
than 30 years after the dwellings have been demolished.

Clearly, what is required for existing council housing is a
regulatory system equivalent to that which was constructed
over a hundred years for the private rented sector (and by
extension, the owner occupied sector). This regulatory
system must include revitalisation but it must also include
clearance. One of the criteria relevant to decisions must be
health. The actual way in which health considerations can be
inserted into such a process will depend on a reorganisation
of the place of community health, in the sense of concern with
the health of the community, both in the National Health
Service and in relation to the operations of local authorities.
In many instances (although clearly not all), attempts at
management solutions to the problems of mass housing 'edifices'
are not appropriate. This is not a criticism of the personnel
involved in intensive management, many of whom do a good job
in difficult circumstances. It is, rather, an assertion that
many of these dwellings, especially those in the form of block
flats, are first and foremost 'edifices' and need to be dealt
with as such.

Action with regard to the organisation of the health services
in relation to housing areas

> Despite many advances in improvements of environ-
> mental control, especially in the more traditional
> sectors i.e. water and air, there is little evidence
> that the physical environment continues to improve;
> rather the reverse with the environment being con-
> tinuously and subtly degraded. (Evidence of the
> Society of Community Medicine to the Royal Commission
> on the National Health Service, 1979)

For anyone with some historical knowledge of the enormous contribution made by preventive medicine to the health of urban
industrial populations, Chapter 14 of the Merrison Report on
the National Health Service (1979) makes disturbing reading.
In it the role of the community physician is defined thus:

> ...those doctors who try to measure and predict the
> health care needs of the population, who plan and
> administer services to meet those needs, and those
> who teach and research in this field. (para. 14.48, p.223)

This is the definition of the Faculty of Community Medicine.
A group of community physicians in the Oxford Region wrote in
similar terms, asserting that the community physician should
be responsible for:

> ...highlighting the health problems of his (sic)
> particular population, for stimulating different
> health professionals to plan their services to
> meet these problems, and for evaluating and monitoring
> the success of these services. (para. 14.50, p. 224)

The tone of the discussion of the role of the community
physician in the Merrison Report suggests that a major problem
is the number of medical officers in post who are employed
solely as administrators (and who are referred to as 'latched
on' doctors - para. 14.48, p. 223), but who have not been
appointed as community physicians. In some respects, there is
a plea for the role of medically expert administrators, the
current role of the district medical officer, which is about
to be subordinated to the 'professional' manager following the
recommendations of the Griffiths Report (1983). There is a
recognition of the potential of epidemology, but very much as
a servant of clinical, curative medicine and with a pronounced
emphasis on the role of individual behaviour (see para. 5.23
p. 47). The discussion supports Blume's (1982) account of
the explanatory model of epidemiology which is cited above,
(p. 47).

All this makes a very recent editorial in the *Journal of
Epidemiology and Community Health* (1984) particularly appo-
site. In: "...and Community Health" the Journal's editors
explain that when the Journal changed its title from *British
Journal of Social and Preventive Medicine:*

> ...we ourselves deliberately did not define what
> we meant by community health but said: "What we have
> in mind at this embryonic stage is not only the study
> of the health state of individuals in a community but
> also the study of the provision of health care, the
> outcome of the treatment of the sick and the prevention
> of disease in the community. We pass the responsibility
> to our contributors over the years to come to
> demonstrate by their publications what the term means
> in practice. (p. 263)

To summarise their account, the editors became concerned
with the diminution of papers:

> ...on the provision of health services..., on social
> conditions leading to ill health or disease, and on the

control or prevention of disease (Ibid)

A special effort to stimulate papers in these areas had
the result that:

> No paper was offered on evaluation of need, none
> on primary health care, none on the social determination
> of disease, none on 'health for all' (Ibid)

The editors concluded:

> But we are worried, even more, that doctors working
> in both academic and service departments of community
> medicine may have lost the fire and spirit that inspired
> the fathers (sic) of social medicine. Epidemiology is a
> difficult and strict discipline which still seems to be
> flourishing. But we hope that our contributors might
> ask more penetrating questions on the health of the
> community, on the provision of care, on the health
> implications of social policy, no matter how embarrass-
> ing the answers might be to their political and
> administrative paymasters. (p. 267)

This interesting editorial makes very clear the decline in
medical research relating to the health of the community as a
whole and/or aggregates within it. The subordination of epidemiology to individualistic conceptions of the determinants of
health and of appropriate health interventions is not just a
matter of explanatory models. It informs research practice
and, most importantly, it informs the current organisation of
health service provision. When beginning the **study** reported
in this book, the authors did not imagine that **one** of the
central conclusions would be to argue for the **return** of the
medical officer of health - but it is.

The subordination of the medical practitioners engaged in
the field of community medicine to a 'curative' dominated
'National Sickness Service' in 1974 was the administrative
culmination of a process which began in the 1950s. In general, as the historical material reviewed in the introduction
to this book shows, attention to the social determinants of
ill health had virtually ceased. Access to curative medicine
under the NHS was seen as the solution to future health problems and the environmental, and especially housing factors
which contributed to ill health were seen as having been
eliminated. Clearly, this was not the case and the need to
re-establish community medicine, concerned with the health of
aggregates rather than individuals, as a central discipline in
social planning is paramount.

The role of the community physician in housing has been
reduced to that of a rationing agent in relation to the
treatment of 'medical priority' cases for rehousing into the
public sector and transfer from undesirable areas within that
public sector. The problem here was clearly identified by
Muir Grey (1978) who pointed out that for individual cases
other than those with restricted mobility seeking transfers
to more accessible dwellings, it is very difficult to assert
that housing transfers will 'improve' health. In other words,
it is difficult to conceptualise better housing for an individual as the appropriate curative treatment for that individual. One might question this, especially in relation to pyscho-
depressive illnesses, and it seems clear that the actions of
some community physicians, (not, it should be stressed, in
Gateshead) in refusing to process such medical priority cases
is, to say the least, high handed.

However, as studies like Bradbury's (1933) demonstrated, it
is entirely possible to conceptualise, and indeed demonstrate,
the efficiency of 'housing' as a treatment for the health of
communities. It seems that the findings of this pilot study
are such as to raise the question of the re-organisation of
community and environmental health in this country. The case
for a partnership between community physician and environmental health officer (not a reverse to the previous medical
domination), located within local authorities (preferably perhaps at a level which does not have housing responsibilities)
and concerned with the effects of the degradation of the
environment on the health of the community seems overwhelming.
There might even be a re-emergence of a series of 'social
epidemiologies' in which the notion of prevention of ill
health associated with factors other than consumption mis-
behaviours of individuals, would be a central objective. The
existence of some sort of wide ranging and informed environmental health service would be a precondition of the proper
organisation of policy under the next heading in this conclusion.

Action with regard to the design, construction and location
of housing in the future

The findings of the study reported in this book cannot be
taken to be simple prescriptions for the design of housing;
including those aspects of site layout which are part of the
urban design process. There is no simple relationship
between housing form and self reported health. Taking account
of the age of the occupants it was clear that the high rise
flats on the Allerdene estate were as 'healthy' as any of the
other areas studied. However, there was a very definite
association between quality, including quality of the environ-

ment in which the housing was located, and health. Allerdene
high rise flats are located in a pleasant suburban environment
and have been well maintained. Access is controlled and
necessary major structural repairs have been executed. Although the unit cost per dwelling is in consequence far higher
than was originally intended, these blocks appear to form a
useful part of the housing stock.

Thus one cannot say that low rise is good and high rise is
bad. Old Fold is low rise and not good. High rise Allerdene
is not bad. Yet it can be argued that there are location,
design and construction conclusions to be drawn from this
study; not in terms of simple prescription of form but rather
in terms of the organisation of processes. What has to be
reiterated here is the importance of a concern for the health
of the future residents at all stages in the design process.
This may seem a contrary thing to say; after all, the historical review of housing and health clearly demonstrated that the
best part of the public sector housing stock is not that which
was built in response to slum clearance motivated by explicit
health concerns, but rather, is that which was the product of
political pressure. Indeed, when housing policy in response
to pressure has been succeeded by policy concerned with
sanitary adequacy, there have been major reductions in the
quality of housing, with detrimental implications for health.
It cannot be said often enough that the best guarantee of
'healthy' housing in the public sector is a powerful and
organised constituency of potential public housing tenants who
are aware of their needs and can exert effective political
pressure.

Thus, in the 1930s the addition to the stock represented by
Old Fold, resulting as it did from slum clearance, was not of
a particularly high quality. However, it was clearly and un-
equivocably better, in terms of its effect on the health of
residents, than the early nineteenth century slums which it
replaced. On the other hand, much of the mass housing built
in the 1960s did not represent an improvement on that which
it replaced. It can, perhaps, be argued that this is
because the health issue was not specifically addressed at
that time. Health had become the province of a curative
health service. If it had not, if the providers of housing
had not dismissed the reservations about density and form
advanced by health orientated critics in the 1950s, then there
would not have been so many dwellings built with totally
inappropriate heating systems and layouts.

The implications to be drawn from this is that those individuals concerned with the quality of housing - environmental
health officers, community physicians (ideally with a

strengthened role akin to the former medical officers of
health) and, most importantly, potential tenants - should have
a direct and major role in the design process. In the 1950s
and 1960s public housing provision involved not merely
increasing concern with costs at the expense of quality
(although the long term costs of low quality housing have
proved to be high) but, in addition, a singular omission of
one of the major objectives of a housing programme - the
improved health of residents. That concern must be returned
to the centre of the process of provision.

This study was designed primarily to investigate the influence of the social aspects of housing design on health. The
survey strategy was designed to elicit people's own views
about their health and their housing. The central concern
was with adequacy at the level of meaning in both methodological and practical terms. The literature reviews conducted
as part of this study demonstrated clearly that, while
designers and constructors became increasingly concerned with
the social implications of their products, there was very
little consideration of the wider, technological elements,
where biological processes of ill health causation may operate directly. Although the impact of materials was not
accessed in any direct fashion by the study reported here,
some mention of potential implications has to be made.

Mass housing was not just an experiment in imposed design.
It also involved a series of innovations in the use of
materials in the construction process. Not all of these were
complete innovations, but in many instances materials which
had been used relatively sparingly, if at all, in the
construction of conventional dwellings now became essential
components of the new stock.

The best known example is asbestos which has been employed
extensively in the insulation of system built accommodation,
often as part of ducted hot air heating systems, a method
which is effective in ensuring the maximum dispersion of
particles in dwellings using that system. The current
complaints about this derive from the industrial campaign
against asbestos in manufacturing. However, asbestos was
not the only new material and many of the others are untested
in terms of their effect on health, as are heating systems
and other aspects of design. The condensation problems which
have been identified extensively in mass housing are one
consequence of the interaction of dwelling design, heating
systems and fuel poverty. It is these aspects of system
built accommodation which were not considered in the original
design and which are still not being considered.

Research into housing and health

Since the beginning of the 1960s there have been enormous changes in the housing system, with the development of mass housing in the public sector and the virtual disappearance of dwellings lacking the basic amenities in the private sectors. Given the significance of these changes, there is a remarkable absence of information about the relationship between health (however defined) and housing. This absence results from changes in the housing system not having been assessed in health terms. The study reported here attempted to redress that omission with a survey of a traditional kind which, while emphasising self reported health, also attempted some 'symptom based' checks. It was always conceived of as a pilot exercise.

While this type of survey has considerable value there is also an important place for other types of research. Together these can provide the basis for methodological triangulation of the nature of relationships between health and housing to provide explanations at the level of both cause and meanings. Thus, there is considerable scope for enthnographic studies of health and housing which expand accounts at the level of meaning and also for more traditional, systematic, biological measurement using some of the procedures employed in occupational medicine which provides explanation at the level of cause. The basic argument of methodological triangulation is that what is told three times is true. The 'health and housing' topic is one in which this general approach to future research would be particularly appropriate.

It is necessary to enter a note of caution about the radical distinction between health defined in terms of the subjective meanings of individuals and in terms of the absence of externally verified pathologies. These two definitions are very different, even though the medical model may be part of the cultural equipment of the individuals constructing social meanings. However, the policy implications for housing and health provision for collectivities, as opposed to intervention in the individual case, may not be different. Indeed, it is the distinction between individual and collective, rather than between health and externally verifiable pathology which is crucial from the point of view of policy formation. This is not to dismiss questions of meaning, but to indicate that the individualistic as well as the mechanical nature of the medical model and its policy consequences should be questioned.

'Mass housing' has proved to be an expensive social disaster, not least, it is suggested, in health terms. The case must be made for the elimination and replacement of this poor quality housing, as well as for the resolution of a range of other housing difficulties of very considerable magnitude. Research, in this context, could be criticised as an excuse for postponing action in the face of evident need, as an 'ideological gloss' on inaction. However, research can often be the stimulus for action. There is currently a prevailing intellectual trend in this country which rejects the potential of informed and systematic intervention for social improvement. This reflects a pessimism of both will and intellect which must be challenged. One way is through the documentation of the nature of contemporary reality. As Alan Walker (1984) argues:

> Objective evidence is an essential feature of
> socialist as much as any other forms of planning,
> It also has an important part to play in putting
> the case for socialism. The deficiencies of
> capitalism are not always as evident as some of those
> on the political left believe them to be... and they
> require detailed exposure. (p. 248)

The types of research advocated above are still at the level of saying 'how things are' in an effort to build up pressure for change. They involve the reconstruction of a social epidemiology of housing and health and the widest possible dissemination of that social epidemiology. However, it should not stop there. If the notion of action research is stripped of its former positivistic assocation with quasi experimental substitutes for social reform, then research can be carried out in conjunction with the implementation of policy, informing it at all stages and allowing for modifications in the light of feedback. However, that is for the future; at this stage the fundamental need is to learn from previous mistakes.

NOTES

(1)   Agreed in principle at a meeting of the Gateshead
      Metropolitan Council's Housing Committee on 7 March
      1985.

Bibliography

AVINERI, S., (1966), The social and political thought of Karl Marx, Oxford University Press : Oxford.

ANESHENSEL, C.S., FRERICHS, R.R., CLARK, A.C., (1981), Family roles and sex differences in depression, Journal of Health and Social Behaviour, 22, pp. 379-393.

BATESON, N., (1984), Data construction in social surveys, Allen and Unwin : London.

BEDALE, C. and FLETCHER, T., (1982), A damp site worse, The Times Health Supplement, 12th February, p. 15.

BLUME, S.G., (1982), Explanation and social policy : the problem of social inequalities in health, Journal of Social Policy, 11, Part 1, pp. 7-31.

BOARD OF TRADE, (1908), Report on rent, wages and prices, HMSO : London.

BRADBURY,F.C.S.(1933), Causal factors in tuberculosis, National Association for the Prevention of Tuberculosis : London.

BROSS, J.D.J., (1958), How to use ridit analysis, Biometrics, 14, pp. 18-38.

BROWN, G.W. and HARRIS, T., (1978), The social origins of depression : a study of psychiatric disorder in women, Tavistock : London.

BYRNE, D.S., (1980), The decline in the standard of council housing in interwar North Shields, in Melling J. (ed.), Housing, social policy and the State, Croom Helm : London.

BYRNE, D.S., (1982), Class and the local State, International Journal of Urban and Regional Research, 6, No.1 pp. 83-98.

141

BYRNE, D.S., and PARSON, D., (1983), The State and the reserve
army, in Anderson, J., Duncan, S. and Hudson, R. (eds.),
Redundant spaces, Academic Press : London.

BYRNE, D.S., (1984), Dublin : a case study of housing and the
residual working class, in International Journal of Urban
and Regional Research, 8, No.3, pp. 402-422.

CENTRAL STATISTICAL OFFICE, (1984), Regional Trends, HMSO :
London.

CHADWICK, E. (1965), Report on the sanitary condition of the
labouring population of Great Britain, (1842), Reprinted
with introduction by M.W. Flinn, Edinburgh University Press
: Edinburgh.

CLANCY, K. and GROVE, W., (1974), Sex differences in mental
illness : an analysis of response bias to self-reports,
American Journal of Sociology, 80, pp. 205-216.

CLEARY, P.D. and MECHANIC, D., (1983) Sex differences in
psychological distress among married people, Journal of
Health and Social Behaviour, 24, pp. 111-121.

COMMUNITY DEVELOPMENT PROJECT : BENWELL, (1976), Slums on the
drawing boards, Benwell Community Development Project.

COMMUNITY DEVELOPMENT PROJECT : NATIONAL, (1977), Whatever
happened to council housing? National Community Development
Project.

COMMUNITY DEVELOPMENT PROJECT : NORTH TYNESIDE, (1977), North
Shields : working class politics and housing 1900-1971,
North Tyneside Community Development Project.

CRONBACH, L.J., (1951), Coefficient alpha and the internal
structure of tests, Psychometrika, 16, pp. 297-334.

CULLINGWORTH, B., (1966), Housing and local government in
England and Wales, Allen and Unwin : London

DAMER, S. (1976), A note on housing allocation, in Edwards, M.
et al. (eds.), Housing and class in Britain, Political
Economy of Housing Workshop : London, pp. 72-74.

DEAN, C., LEE, P.N., TODD, G.F., WICKEN, A.J., SPARKS, D.M.,
(1978), Factors relating to respiratory and cardio-vascular
symptoms in the United Kingdom, Journal of Epidemiology and
Community Health, 32, pp. 260-266.

DENNIS, N., (1970), People and planning, Faber : London.

DENNIS, N., (1972), Public participation and planners'
blight, Faber : London

DEPARTMENT OF COMMUNITY MEDICINE : ST THOMAS'S HOSPITAL
MEDICAL SCHOOL, (undated), National study of the health and
growth of schoolchildren.

DEPARTMENT OF EMPLOYMENT, (1981), Department of Employment
Gazette, June.

DEPARTMENT OF EMPLOYMENT, (1983), Department of Employment
Gazette, June

DEPARTMENT OF THE ENVIRONMENT, (1978) English House Condition Survey 1976, Part 1. Report of the physical condition
survey, Housing Survey Report No. 10, HMSO : London

DEPARTMENT OF THE ENVIRONMENT, (1979a), English House Condit-
ion Survey 1976, Part 2. Report of the social survey,
Housing Survey Report No. 11, HMSO : London.
DEPARTMENT OF THE ENVIRONMENT, (1979b), National Dwelling and
Housing Survey, HMSO : London.
DEPARTMENT OF THE ENVIRONMENT, (1980a), National Dwelling and
Housing Survey, Phases II and III, HMSO : London.
DEPARTMENT OF THE ENVIRONMENT, (1980b), Housing Development
Directorate Occasional Paper 3/80, Vol. 1 : General find-
ings, HMSO : London.
DEPARTMENT OF THE ENVIRONMENT, (1980c), Housing Development
Directorate Occasional Paper 4/80, An investigation of
difficult-to-let housing, Vol.2: Case studies of postwar
estates, HMSO : London.
DEPARTMENT OF THE ENVIRONMENT, (1980d), Housing Development
Directorate Occasional Paper 5/80, An investigation into
difficult-to-let housing, Vol.3: Case studies of prewar
estates, HMSO : London.
DEPARTMENT OF THE ENVIRONMENT, (1981), Priority estates,
HMSO : London.
DEPARTMENT OF THE ENVIRONMENT, (1982), English House Condition
Survey 1981, Part 1 : Report of the physical condition sur-
vey, Housing Survey Report No. 12, HMSO : London.
DEPARTMENT OF THE ENVIRONMENT, (1983), English House Condition
Survey 1981, Part 2 : Report of the interview and local
authority survey, Housing Survey Report No. 13, HMSO :
London.
DEPARTMENT OF HEALTH AND SOCIAL SECURITY, (1980), Inequalities
in health : Report of a research working group (Chairman,
Sir Douglas Black), DHSS : London.
DOHRENWEND, B. and DOHRENWEND B., (1976), Sex differences and
psychiatric disorders, American Journal of Psychology, 81,
pp. 1447-1454.
DONNISON, D. and UNGERSON, C., (1982), Housing policy, Penguin
: Middlesex.
DOYAL, L., (1979), The political economy of health, Pluto :
London.
DUNLEAVY, P., (1981), Mass housing in Britain, Oxford Univer-
sity Press : Oxford.
ENGELS, F., (1958), (translated and edited by Henderson, W.O.
and Chaloner, W.H.), The condition of the working class in
England, Blackwell : Oxford.
EVERITT, B.S., (1974), Cluster analysis, Heinemann : London.
FAMILY SERVICE UNITS, (1983), Homes fit for people, Family
Service Units Discussion Paper, Family Service Units :
London.
FANNING, D.M., (1967), Families in flats, British Medical
Journal, 4, pp. 383-386.

143

FORREST, R., (1982), Social implications of council house sales, in English, J. (ed.), The future of council housing, Croom Helm : London.

FORREST, R. and MURIE, A., (1983), Residualisation and council housing, Journal of Social Policy, 12, Part 4, pp. 453-468.

FOX, J., and GOLDBLATT, P., (1978), Household mortality from the OPCS longitudinal study, Population Trends, HMSO : London.

FRANEY, R., (1981), Would you live here?, Roof, July/August, pp. 10-12.

FRIEDMAN, A., (1977) Industry and labour, Macmillan : London.

FRIEND, A. and METCALF, A., (1981) Slump city, Pluto : London.

GAULDIE, E., (1974), Cruel habitations : a history of working-class housing 1780-1918, Allen and Unwin : London.

GENERAL REGISTER OFFICE, (1964), Census 1961 England and Wales, Housing Tables Part 1, Buildings, dwellings and households, HMSO : London.

GIBSON, I., (1981), Class, health and profit, University of East Anglia : Norwich.

GILBERT, G.N., (1983), Modelling society : an introduction to log-linear analysis for social researchers, Allen and Unwin : London.

GIRT, J.L., (1972), Simple chronic bronchitis and urban ecological structure, in McGlasher, N.D. (ed.), Medical geography, Methuen : London.

GITTUS, E., (1976), Flats, families and the under fives, Routledge and Kegan Paul, London.

GREAT BRITAIN NHS MANAGEMENT INQUIRY TEAM, (1983), NHS Management Inquiry Report, (Leader of the Inquiry, R. Griffiths), DHSS : Stanmore.

GUILDFORD, J.P., (1965), Fundamental statistics in psychology and education, McGraw Hill : London.

HANNAY, D.R., (1979), The symptom iceberg : a study of community health, Routledge and Kegan Paul : London.

HANSARD., (1929-30), House of Commons Debate, 237, p. 2014

HARRISON, P., (1983), Living in the inner city, Penguin : London.

HAWTHORNE, V.M. and FRY, J.S., (1978), Smoking and health : the association between smoking behaviour, total mortality and cardio-respiratory disease in Western Scotland, Journal of Epidemiology and Community Health, 32, pp. 260-266.

HELLEVIK, O., (1984), Introduction to causal analysis, Allen and Unwin : London.

HIRD, J.F.B., (1966), Planning for a new community, The Journal of the Royal College of General Practitioners, 12, Supplement No. 1, pp. 33-41.

HOURIHAN, K., (1984), Residential satisfaction, neighbourhood
    attributes and personal characteristics : an exploratory
    path analysis; in Cork, Ireland, Environment and planning A,
    16, pp. 425-436.
INEICHEN, B., (1983), Council housing and disadvantage; the
    allocation of council housing and its relation to social
    stratification, in Brown, M., The structure of disadvantage,
    Heinemann : London.
INTERNATIONAL CLASSIFICATION OF HEALTH PROBLEMS IN PRIMARY
    HEALTH CARE, (1979), (Revised edition), Oxford University
    Press : Oxford.
JONES, C., (1967), The removal of areas of twilight housing,
    Living in Britain, RIBA Conference, July, p. 4.
JOURNAL OF EPIDEMIOLOGY AND COMMUNITY HEALTH, (1984), '...and
    community health' (editorial) 38, pp. 263-264.
JOWELL, R. and AIREY, C., (1984), British social attitudes:
    the 1984 report, Gower Publishing Company Limited :
    Aldershot.
KESSLER, R.C. and McRAE, J.A., (1981), Trends in the relation-
    ship between sex and psychological distress, American
    Sociological Review, 46, pp. 443-452.
LAMBERT, P.M. and REID, D.D., (1970), Smoking, air pollution
    and bronchitis in Britain, Lancet, 1, No. 7652, pp. 853-857.
LIEBERMAN, B. (ed.), (1971), Contemporary problems in social
    statistics : a book of readings for the social sciences,
    Oxford University Press : Oxford.
LITTLEWOOD, J. and TINKER, A., (1981), Families in flats,
    HMSO : London.
M'GONIGLE, G.C.M., (1933), Proceedings of the Royal Society
    of Medicine, 26, p. 67
MANDERS, F.W.D., (1973), A history of Gateshead, Gateshead
    Metropolitan Borough Council.
MARSH, C., (1982), The survey method, Allen and Unwin :
    London.
MARTIN, A.F., (1967), Environment, housing and health, Urban
    Studies, 4, No. 1, pp. 1-21.
MEDICAL OFFICER OF HEALTH FOR GATESHEAD, (1911), Annual Report
MEDICAL OFFICER OF HEALTH FOR GATESHEAD, (1912), Annual Report
MEDICAL OFFICER OF HEALTH FOR GATESHEAD, (1930), Annual Report
MEDICAL OFFICER OF HEALTH FOR GATESHEAD, (1933), Annual Report
MEDICAL RESEARCH COUNCIL, (undated) Questionnaire on
    respiratory symptoms 1976, Medical Research Council :
    London.
MELLING, J., (1980), Housing, social policy and the State,
    Croom Helm : London.
MERRETT, S., (1979), State housing in Britain, Routledge and
    Kegan Paul : London.
MINISTRY OF HOUSING AND LOCAL GOVERNMENT, (1956), Report of
    the Ministry, 1955, Cmd. 9876, HMSO : London.

MINISTRY OF HOUSING AND LOCAL GOVERNMENT, (1961), Homes for today and tomorrow : Report of a Sub-Committee of the Central Housing Advisory Committee, (Chairman, Sir Parker Morris), HMSO : London.

MORGAN, M. and CHENN, S., (1983), ACORN GROUP, Social class and child health, Journal of Epidemiology and Community Health, 31, pp. 196-203.

MUIR-GREY, J., (1978), Housing, health and illness, British Medical Journal, 2, pp. 100-101.

MURRAY, J., DUNN, G., TARPOLSKY, S., (1982), Self-assessment of health : an exploration of the effects of physical and psychological symptoms, Psychological Medicine, 12, pp. 371-378.

NAVARRO, V., (1978), Class struggle, the State and medicine, Martin Robertson : London.

NICHOLS, T., (1979), Social class, official, sociological and Marxist, in Irvine, J. et al (eds.), Demystifying social statistics, Pluto : London.

OFFICE OF POPULATION CENSUSES AND SURVEYS, (1980), Classification of occupations and coding index, HMSO : London.

OFFICE OF POPULATION CENSUSES AND SURVEYS, (1983), Census 1981 : Housing and households, HMSO : London.

OFFICE OF POPULATION CENSUSES AND SURVEYS, (1984), General Household Survey 1982, HMSO : London.

ORMANDY, D., (1981), Overcrowding, Roof, March/April, pp. 11-12.

PAYNE, G. and PAYNE J., (1977), Housing pathways and stratification, Journal of Social Policy, 6, Part 2, pp. 129-156.

PEET, R., (1975), Inequality and poverty : a Marxist - Geographic theory, Annals of the Association of American Geographers, 65, No. 4, pp. 564-571.

PHILLIPS, D. and SEGAL, B., (1969), Sexual states and psychiatric symptoms, American Sociological Review, 34, pp. 58-72.

PIKE, L., (1981), Morbidity and environment in an urban general practice in Birmingham, Birchfield Medical Centre and Department of Engineering Production, University of Birmingham.

RAWLINSON, R., (1850), Report on a preliminary inquiry into the borough of Gateshead, Board of Health.

RICHMAN, N., (1974), The effects of housing on pre-school children and their mothers, Developments in Medicine and Child Neurology, 16, pp. 53-58.

ROGERS, F.W., (1971), Gateshead and the public health act of 1848, Archaelogica Aeliana, 4th series, 49, pp. 153-186.

ROYAL COMMISSION ON THE HOUSING OF THE WORKING CLASSES, (1885), Parlimentary papers 1884-1885, Vol. XXX, HMSO : London.

ROYAL COMMISSION ON THE NATIONAL HEALTH SERVICE, (1979),
Report (Chairman, Sir Alec Merrison), Cmnd. 7615, HMSO :
London.

SCHUESSLER, K., (1972), Analyzing social data : a statistical
orientation, Houghton : Boston.

SIMON OF WYTHENSHAWE, (1929), How to abolish the slums,
London.

SWENARTON, M., (1981), Homes fit for heroes, Heinemann :
London.

TAYLOR, P.J., (1979), 'Difficult to let', 'difficult to live
in' and sometimes 'difficult to get out of' : an essay on
the provision of council housing, with special reference
to Killingworth, Environment and Planning A, 11, pp. 1305-
1320.

THOMPSON, E.P., (1978), The poverty of theory, Merlin :
London.

TOWNSEND, P., (1973), Everyone his own home, Royal Institute
of British Architects Journal, January.

TOWNSEND, P., (1979), Poverty in the United Kingdom, Penguin
: London.

TUCKER, J., (1966), Honourable estates, Gollancz : London.

WALKER, A., (1984), Social planning, Blackwell : Oxford.

WILLIAMS, R., (1981), Politics and letters, Verso : London.

ZELLER, R.A. and CARMINES, E.G., (1980), Measurement in the
social sciences, Cambridge University Press : Cambridge.

Index